Herbal Tea

OVER 150 EASY TO MAKE HEALTH HERBAL TEA
RECIPES FOR MORE THAN 30 COMMON AILMENTS

HEATHER DALE

Medical Advice Disclaimer

Contents

Introduction

Herbal teas and herbal medicine have a long-established tradition in almost all cultures worldwide.

This history is both moving and vibrant, and using herbs as medicine is again returning to us after thousands of years and hundreds of years of persecution. Herbal medicine is something I love and have written much about, but sometimes it is better to have the essential items without pages on the why's and the where's!

This short book is, therefore, about something other than the rich history of herbal medicine and the many uses, properties, and actions that a herb has. It is to provide an easy-to-use recipe book of herbal teas that explains why each herb is suitable for a particular ailment. Its purpose is to be as practical as possible.

Herbal teas are remarkably easy to prepare, a cost-effective remedy, and in many cases, you will already have the herbs on your kitchen shelf.

Tea allows you to benefit from its medicinal properties and enjoy its soothing effects on the entire body, mind, and soul.

Like all herbs, you should always check with a medical professional before use, especially if you have a pre-existing condition or are using any medication. Herbs can interact with these and even have the opposite effect to that of which you are aiming for, so remember to respect these plants; they may taste great but can be powerful!

In the following chapters, I will explain how to make teas, then outline some other uses and some of the most common herbs and dosages before listing over 150 tea recipes you can prepare. There are 4 or 5 recipes for each condition, which means that you can find the one that works best for you - we are all different, and we will all have our preferred tea.

I have also added information on body systems - even a brief understanding of these is valuable, and I have only included an overview in the following pages.

CHAPTER 1

Preparing your tea and other uses

What to Consider Before Creating Herbal Teas

As fun and healthy as it is to create your own medicinal teas, it's important to consider a few things before you get started. These will help you establish your priorities as well as create a routine that is not only safe but also enjoyable.

Some things you want to think about include the following:

- Are you or the one being treated on any prescribed medications or supplements? This is due to the possibility of negative reactions when combining these treatments.
- What exactly is the ailment that requires treatment?
- Which organs will benefit?
- Are you trying to stimulate any specific emotions?
- Keep the energetics of the condition and person in mind. Cold people and conditions require warming herbs, whereas warm people and conditions require cooling herbs.

Remember that there is no one way to do something. It is your creation, and as long as done correctly and with caution, you can experiment and make it your own and try not to focus on only treating one symptom. As your herbal knowledge grows, try creating blends that have multiple benefits including treating the desired issue.

Herbal teas are only going to fix certain problems and you or the person being treated may need to make some lifestyle changes like introducing exercise and a healthy diet.

PREPARATION

To prepare fresh herbs for herbal tea, follow these steps:

- Rinse the herbs thoroughly to remove any dirt or debris.
- Remove any tough stems or wilted leaves.
- Chop or tear the herbs into small pieces to help release their flavors.
- Place the herbs in a cup or teapot.
- Pour boiling water over the herbs.
- Cover the cup or teapot and let the herbs steep for five to 10 minutes, depending on the strength desired.
- Strain the herbs out of the water before drinking.

Steeping time

Below is a general rule of thumb for the most common herbal teas in terms of how long to steep your herbs. You can soak for longer to get a more robust flavor and sometimes a more potent effect.

- Flowers - 5 to 10 minutes
- Seeds - 10 minutes
- Bark - 10 to 15 minutes

If you prefer a stronger herbal tea, you can use more herbs or steep the herbs for a longer period of time. It's important to note that different herbs may have different preparation methods and recommended dosages.

Preparation methods

There are several different preparation methods for herbal tea and the following pages focus on infusions, but here are some of the other popular options:

- Infusion: To prepare an infusion, add one to two teaspoons of dried herbs or two to three teaspoons of fresh herbs to a cup of boiling water. Cover the cup and let the herbs steep for five to 10 minutes, depending on the strength desired. Strain the herbs out of the water before drinking.
- Decoction: To prepare a decoction, add one to two teaspoons of dried herbs or two to three teaspoons of fresh herbs to a cup of water in a small saucepan. Bring the water to a boil, then reduce the heat and simmer for 10 to 15 minutes. Strain the herbs out of the water before drinking.
- Cold brew: To prepare a cold brew, add one to two teaspoons of dried herbs or two to three teaspoons of fresh herbs to a cup of cold water. Cover the cup and let the herbs steep in the refrigerator for several hours or overnight. Strain the herbs out of the water before drinking.
- Tincture: To prepare a tincture, add one to two teaspoons of dried herbs or two to three teaspoons of fresh herbs to a cup of alcohol, such as vodka or brandy. Cover the cup and let the herbs steep in a cool, dark place for several weeks. Strain the herbs out of the alcohol before drinking. Tinctures are usually taken by the drop, rather than by the cup.

Medical Decoctions

Decoctions are generally the preparation method for denser plant products like stems, bark, roots, and seeds. Many of the desired nutrients are harder to extract than with delicate plant products, so they cannot be drawn out simply using the steeping method. This is why they are best to be simmered in the water to ensure the necessary constituents are effectively extracted - like the iron and copper found in red clover blossoms or the silica found in oat straw. These components cannot be steeped out so they need the decocting method.

How to Decoct Herbs

In a pot or saucepan, add three tablespoons of your desired herb to a quart of cold water. Heat this water at a very low temperature and be sure to cover the pot. Remember that simmering on the heat will likely reduce the amount of water you're left with, so don't be alarmed when you return and find the water is less. Allow simmering to continue between 20 to 45 minutes. You can now strain your water into a jar. Larger batches of decoctions may last as long as a week in the fridge. You can either add a bit of your decoction to juices or infuse with water.

Dosages

The dosage of how frequently you're going to use any of the methods below will depend on the ailment and whether or not your symptoms are improving. It's highly advisable not to use any remedies in place of prescribed medication or in conjunction with prescribed meds as they may interfere with its effectiveness. Nevertheless, if you're treating certain ailments with herbal teas and are unsure of the dosage, let's have a look at some standard recommendations.

How many cups of tea you should drink depends on the condition being treated. Chronic illnesses may necessitate a cup of the herbal tea remedy at least three times a day, whereas severe conditions may call for one cup every 2 hours of awake time.

It's important to use herbal tea remedies for a week before reassessing your condition and ascertaining whether or not you need to continue or seek help.

You may also want to pulse your doses which basically means taking the tea for a certain period of time and then taking a break before continuing again.

How this will look is, if you're using it for 6 days, you would then not use it for one day, and if you're using it for 10 days, you would not use it for 3 days.

OTHERS WAYS TO BENEFIT FROM HERBAL TEA

Herbal teas contain a wide range of essential nutrients that are also water-soluble, such as enzymes, saponins, carbohydrates, and more.

Though teas are commonly used as a nutritious beverage, many people underestimate their versatility. This herbal remedy is not only for cleansing your insides and preventing internal complications but can also be applied to the skin in a variety of ways.

Below I have included just some examples of the other ways that you can use your herbal tea.

Steam your face

Facial steams are not only useful to help treat certain skin problems but are also great for simply relieving facial tension, detoxing your skin, and improving circulation which will leave you with an undeniable glow. This kind of treatment is recommended at least once a week (you can do it more if you feel it's necessary). You're going to ensure your hair is tied and won't get in the way and then wash your face as you'd normally do. Then, add about two tablespoons of herbs to a quart of boiling water in a glass bowl and hold your head directly above it. It's important to use a rag or towel to cover your head so that the steam remains inside. You may have to lift the towel every now and then as the steam can be quite intense, but you want to inhale the steam for about 5 to 7 minutes for optimal results. You can pat your face dry with the towel or splash with some cold water after.

- **Lavender** – Soothing and calming. Relieves itching, is astringent, and anti-bacterial.
- **Calendula** – Helpful for those with eczema and psoriasis. It is anti-inflammatory, astringent and anti-microbial.
- **Chamomile** – Helpful for dry, irritated skin. It is anti-inflammatory, anti-bacterial, and has anti-viral properties.
- **White Willow Bark** – calms redness and inflammation and has anti-microbial and anti-fungal properties.
- **Peppermint** – Refreshing, anti-inflammatory and anti-microbial and is helpful for dull, oily, or irritated skin.
- You can use these herbs for most skin conditions.

Baths

There are different kinds of baths, all with their own unique therapeutic benefits. You may not have time for a full body bath all the time, which is why there are handbaths and footbaths. Each method provides you with the benefits of the tea you're using so don't feel bad when you can only get to a footbath one week and a handbath the following week.

Handbaths

Your hands consist of many nerve endings. Treating these nerve endings can have countless benefits like improved circulation, colds, arthritis, and flu. It can also relieve aches in the hand and symptoms of eczema. Make at least two quarts of tea in a bowl and soak your hands in it (as soon as the temperature is manageable). You can do so for about 5 to 10 minutes.

Sitz baths

This kind of bath can be taken in a regular-sized bath or even in a small basin. Warm sitz baths are good for combating congestion, relieving pains, such as hemorrhoid pain and gynecological issues, and improving circulation to the pelvic area. You'll have to pour your herbal tea mixture into the tub or basin and soak in it for about three minutes. It's best if your entire pelvic section is immersed in the herbal mixture. Cold or cool sitz baths are also good to try as it assists with menstrual cramps, pelvic inflammatory disease, congestion of the spleen or liver and improves functions of the bowel and lower organs, hemorrhoids, and general back issues.

Some people have actually said that alternating between hot and cool sitz baths offers more significant healing and is a great way to remove toxins and draw in nutrients.

You should always start with the hot bath and then move to the cold. So soak in the hot sitz bath for three minutes and in the cool bath for two minutes. This process can be followed three times for the most effective results. It's important to keep warm once you've finished the entire process.

Witch Hazel is believed to soothe hemorrhoids - it is an astringent and anti-inflammatory.

Lavender is great to add to your bath - its calming property is good for anxiety, insomnia and depression - and it smells great!

You can mix these with **Calendula, Yarrow** and **Uva Ursi** - traditionally used to treat any bladder-related infections including Urinary tract infections.

Add you mix to a muslin bag before adding to your bath.

Footbaths

Our feet also contain various nerve endings which is why footbaths can be so helpful to relieve calluses, aching feet, varicose veins, and leg cramps and even remove bad odors. Much like with sitz baths, footbaths don't necessarily have to be hot; you can also benefit from a cold or cool footbath. The ideal foot bath is made with four quarts of herbal tea and placed in a basin where you'll be soaking your feet. If you notice the first symptoms of an approaching cold, you can take a footbath to relieve congestion, headache, and sore throats. Remember to rinse your feet with cold water when you're done, dry them properly, and keep them warm with socks.

Full body baths

This kind of bath has a range of ways you can enjoy absorbing the nutrients from your teas into your skin. You can add the herbs to a sock or muslin, which can be tied to the faucet as you let two quarts of water run through it into the tub, or simply allow it to soak in the water with you. Alternatively, you can make the tea in a container before adding it to your bath water. Your skin isn't the only thing that'll benefit, since you'll be inhaling the nutrient-rich steam too. It's also good for soothing certain skin conditions, and most teas are safe for use in children. Doing so before their bedtime will improve the chances of a good night's sleep.

Examples are:

- Lavender (relaxing - add mint, lemon or rose)
- Chamomile (soothing and relaxing)

Hair washes

This isn't only ideal for a personal pampering session but also helps for treating oily hair, dandruff, dry scalp, and even balding. You're going to use four heaped teaspoons of herbs for every quart of water. Stir it well and allow it to steep for about an hour, ensuring that it's covered. Strain the herbs out and add them to a spray or squeeze bottle for easy application. For extra strength and shine, add a tablespoon of apple cider vinegar to the mixture and begin applying it to your hair. You should focus on applying it to your scalp and eventually saturating your entire head. Allow the mixture to dry on your hair naturally. Herbs for your hair include:

- Rosemary - hair growth, anti-dandruff, itchy scalp
- Nettle - hair growth and scalp health
- Horsetail - scalp health, anti-dandruff, reduces oil in oily hair
- Chamomile - boost shine and hydration
- Lavender - itchy scalp and dandruff

Mouthwashes

The ideal herbs for mouthwash are lemon balm, licorice, plantain, calendula, echinacea, sage, chamomile, or thyme. The preparation is simple because you'll simply be making an infusion and allowing it to cool off before using it to gargle with. The ideal period to continue this process is for about 10 minutes.

Eye drops

Recent years have increased our time in front of cellphones and computers, and this remedy is perfect for treating tired, sore, infected, or inflamed eyes.

The recommended herbs for making eye washes are fenugreek, plantain, basil, chamomile, rosemary, elderflower, thyme, raspberry leaf, fennel, calendula, and red clover blossoms. Since you're making eye drops, you need to make the mixture much weaker than you would for ingestion or for your baths. For every cup of water, add a small teaspoon of herbs, and simmer on extremely low heat for approximately 10 minutes.

For straining, ensure that the strainer is efficient enough to remove even the smallest particles as you do not want any of them getting into your eyes. Now pour the strained mixture into a well-sterilized eyecup and drop it into our eyes. Be sure to blink so that the mixture washes the entire eye and not just one section. You can do this daily to reduce the chances of bacteria getting into your eyes.

Steam inhalations

You'll generally resort to steam inhalations when you need relief from respiratory problems like nasal congestion, bronchitis, coughs, asthma, sinusitis, or to loosen phlegm. Aromatic herbs like oregano, yarrow, thyme, and mint are best suited for this method. You're going to boil one quart of water, and once boiling, remove it from the heat and pour into a glass bowl. Now add four heaped teaspoons of one of the mentioned herbs to the water, lean your head over the bowl, and cover your head with a rag or towel to get as much steam as possible. You can do this for about 7 minutes, but remember to let some cool air in every now and then if the steam is too overwhelming.

Compresses

These can also be used either hot or cold and are useful for a variety of ailments. This basically involves soaking a face cloth or towel in your desired tea mixture, wringing the water out and applying the cloth to the necessary area. Muslin bags are also a good choice. Compresses are ideal for treating skin problems like rashes and infections, improving circulation, relieving pain, reducing inflammation, and more. Cold compresses are best suited for reducing swelling of inflamed areas, and the recommended herb to use is peppermint. Just be sure to keep the problem area warm after treatment, as this prevents feeling too cold. Hot compresses are best suited for arthritic pains, back pains, and sore throats and are commonly used with hot ginger tea. When using a hot compress, you may want to follow up with a brief cool compress.

CHAPTER 2
What are Herbal teas

Herbal teas are perhaps better described as herbal infusions or "tisanes." They are made with hot water and parts of plants or herbs such as leaves, bark, flowers, and roots. Additionally, they don't contain caffeine. This makes them different from other teas, such as black, green, and white, all made from the tea plant *Camellia sinensis.*

The preparation for almost all herbal teas is remarkably similar.

Herbal tea can boost you in many ways because it is a medicine for the body, mind, and spirit. The more intention you bring to the process, the more it will benefit you.

As herbal teas are preventative medicine, they can (and should) be taken regularly, even daily. It is very easy to research your own mixtures of herbs and roots, to improve taste or to provide different health benefits.

For example, Peppermint tea is used for an upset stomach, headache, irritable bowel syndrome, and even breathing problems.

Chamomile tea is used for relaxation and, famously, to help you fall asleep. But, many people believe that lavender is more effective. It helps with ease upset stomach, gas, diarrhea, insomnia, and anxiety as well as easing stomach upsets, gas, and diarrhea.

Rooibos tea comes from a plant native to South Africa. It is known for its antioxidants and is believed to boost the immune system and help prevent cancer. It may also be good for your heart and help fight diabetes.

Echinacea tea or coneflower is a well-known cold remedy that boosts the immune system and may help with the flu. Don't drink this tea or use Echinacea if you're pregnant, have allergies, or have asthma, and it can also affect how well certain drugs work.

Milk Thistle and dandelion tea are used to help with liver and gallbladder problems. The main ingredient in milk thistle is silymarin, which may ease the symptoms of hepatitis C.

They are surprisingly easy to create. First, find a blend that works and mix the ingredients (dried) in a bowl. Then store them safely. When you want to brew your tea, take one teaspoon, and add it to a cup of boiled water. If you want a stronger taste, you can use a larger spoonful of herbs or less water — the longer you steep the herbal mixture in the water, the more compounds are extracted.

Teas involve pouring water over either fresh leaves, processed leaves, or flowers of a tea plant. In some cases, you can make tea from certain roots, like valerian or ginger, which don't include any leaves; however, the method of preparation is like that of teas.

It's generally a good rule of thumb to avoid using any aluminum tools and containers with all these preparations. Teas don't usually require much time to strew but it all depends on you and how potent you'd like your mixture to be, as well as what kind of tea you're preparing. The longer you leave the tea to brew, the stronger it will be.

THE STANDARD FORMULA

In the case of fresh herbs two teaspoons should be enough or one teaspoon when using dried herbs.

In general when you see the term 'one part' or 'part' it refers to either the fresh or dried herbs. It's important to remember that the steeping time will vary depending on the density of whatever herb you're using.

For instance, barks and roots are best when steeped overnight, flowers are good within two hours, leaves require about four hours, and seeds can be steeped for about an hour.

Steeping time

Below is a general rule of thumb for the most common herbal teas in terms of how long to steep your herbs for. You can steep for longer to get a stronger flavor and sometimes a stronger effect.

- Flowers - 5 to 10 minutes
- Seeds - 10 minutes
- Bark - 10 to 15 minutes

How Long Will Your Tea Last?

This depends on the type of tea, fermentation method, and whether or not the leaves are undamaged. If a tea leaf is still very much intact and has been well fermented, it will last longer. to get the longest shelf life out of your teas, be sure to store them in airtight containers away from water, heat, and light.

Benefits of Herbal Tea

Below is a brief list of some of the best herbs for herbal teas and their specific uses. You can mix more than one, for example stress and healthy skin or stress and improved sleep using the standard herbal tea formula.

Healthy Skin

- rose hip
- raspberry leaf
- milk thistle
- burdock root
- licorice root
- nettles

Stress Relievers

- chamomile
- holy basil (also known as Tulsi)
- damiana
- lavender
- skullcap

Healthy Digestion

- licorice root
- fennel
- lemon balm
- peppermint
- slippery elm
- marshmallow root
- ginger

Healthy Immune

- elderberry
- rose hips
- echinacea
- mullein
- licorice root
- turmeric
- ginger

Improved Sleep

- wood betony
- chamomile
- lavender
- skullcap
- passionflower
- valerian root

Increased Energy

- ginseng
- licorice root
- schisandra berry
- eleuthero

Example of popular herbal teas

Some of the most popular herbal teas include:

1. Chamomile tea - made from the dried flowers of the Chamomile plant, it has a sweet, apple-like taste and is often used as a natural sleep aid.
2. Peppermint tea - made from the leaves of the peppermint plant, it has a refreshing, minty taste and is often used to help with digestion.
3. Green tea - made from the leaves of the Camellia sinensis plant, it has a light, grassy taste and is high in antioxidants.
4. Ginger tea - made from the root of the ginger plant, it has a spicy, warming taste and is often used to help with nausea and digestion.
5. Echinacea tea - made from the Echinacea plant, it has a sweet, slightly bitter taste and is often used to help boost the immune system.
6. Rooibos tea - made from the leaves of the Rooibos plant, it has a slightly sweet, nutty taste and is high in antioxidants.
7. Lemon balm tea - made from the leaves of the lemon balm plant, it has a light, lemony taste and is often used to help with anxiety and stress.
8. Dandelion tea - made from the leaves and roots of the dandelion plant, it has a slightly bitter taste and is often used to help with liver function and digestion.

Now that you have an understanding of what benefits herbs can offer, in the next chapter we will highlight some of the most common and 'safest' herbs as well as some herbs to avoid (unless you know what you are doing or are under professional supervision). Once again a reminder not to use herbs if you have any pre-existing condition or are taking any other medication and you should always consult with a physician before using herbal remedies - herbs are powerful.

.

CHAPTER 3

Herbs to use and herbs to avoid

It is always useful to know how else a herb could be used and applied and here we provide a summary of the most common herbs and uses. We will also mention herbs to avoid as this is equally useful!

SAFEST HERBS

Here is a list of 20 safe herbs that you can use in tea or other herbal preparations:

1. Chamomile: Chamomile is a calming herb that has been used for centuries to help with sleep and relaxation.
2. Peppermint: Peppermint is a refreshing herb that has been used to help with digestion and headaches.
3. Ginger: Ginger is a warming herb that has been used to help with nausea and inflammation.
4. Turmeric: Turmeric is a potent antioxidant that has been used to help with inflammation and pain.
5. Lavender: Lavender is a calming herb that has been used to help with sleep and relaxation.
6. Rosemary: Rosemary is an herb that has been used to help with concentration and memory.
7. Echinacea: Echinacea is an herb that has been used to help with the common cold and other respiratory infections.
8. Basil: Basil is an herb that has been used to help with digestion and to add flavor to food.
9. Thyme: Thyme is an herb that has been used to help with respiratory issues and as a natural expectorant.
10. Calendula: Calendula is an herb that has been used to help with skin irritation and inflammation.
11. Dandelion: Dandelion is an herb that has been used to help with digestion and as a natural diuretic.
12. Hops: Hops is an herb that has been used to help with sleep and relaxation.
13. Lemon balm: Lemon balm is an herb that has been used to help with sleep and to reduce anxiety.

14. Marjoram: Marjoram is an herb that has been used to help with digestion and to reduce muscle spasms.
15. Nettle: Nettle is an herb that has been used to help with allergy symptoms and as a natural diuretic.
16. Red clover: Red clover is an herb that has been used to help with menopausal symptoms and as a natural expectorant.
17. Sage: Sage is an herb that has been used to help with memory and to reduce hot flashes.
18. St. John's wort: St. John's wort is an herb that has been used to help with depression and anxiety.
19. Valerian: Valerian is an herb that has been used to help with sleep and anxiety.
20. Yarrow: Yarrow is an herb that has been used to help with skin irritation and to reduce inflammation.

When you are selecting your herbs a great way to note how, and if you want to use them, is to use a simple journal and takes notes. Below is an example using some of the most common herbs that includes what to be aware of when you are considering their use and it underscores that if you have any preexisting conditions you really must consult with your physician.

Catnip

- **Precautions**: Excessive use can lead to vomiting. Not recommended for use in pregnant women.
- **Topical uses**: Hair wash for the irritated scalp, enema for cleaning out the colon, steam inhalations for nasal congestion, poultice or compress for treating bruises, toothache, hemorrhoids, and muscle sprains. Can also be used as an eyewash for bloodshot eyes or allergy-induced eye irritations.
- **Uses in teas**: Treats digestive problems like indigestion, diarrhea, gas, muscle spasms, abdominal pains, as well as cold and flu-related issues like smallpox, chickenpox, bronchitis, mumps, measles, and insomnia, hyperactivity, and anxiety.

Chamomile

- **Precautions**: Roman chamomile has a greater chance of causing an allergic reaction than German chamomile. People who are sensitive to ragweed may have severe reactions to this plant.
- **Topical uses**: Can be used as a mouthwash to treat or prevent gingivitis, eye drops for treating conjunctivitis, compress for the treatment of wounds, eczema, psoriasis, burns, insect bites and stings, skin ulcers, baths for treating hemorrhoids, dry skin, or relieving stress or cranky children
- **Uses in teas**: Relieves digestive problems like irritable bowel syndrome, indigestion, gut inflammation, gas, and intestinal cramps and soothes hyperactivity, neural fatigue, restlessness, and insomnia.

Cinnamon

- **Precautions**: Not suitable for use when suffering from fever, blood in your urine, excessive dryness, dry stools, hemorrhoids, or while nursing or pregnant
- **Topical uses**: Baths can soothe aching muscles and treat chills, footbaths for fungal infection, mouthwash to eliminate bad breath, and steam inhalations for colds, sore throats, and coughs.
- **Uses in teas**: Good for reducing cholesterol and blood sugar, strengthening and improving digestive tract functions and heart health, and can also treat diarrhea.

Dandelion

- **Precautions**: Professional medical advice or guidance is advised for people with gallstones or structured bile ducts. Excessive use may cause allergic reactions, abdominal problems, heartburn, nausea, or loose stools. Possible worsened symptoms in gastric hyperacidity.
- **Topical uses**: Used as a wash for treating fungal infections
- •**Uses in teas**: Used for treating jaundice in infants, increasing breast milk supply in nursing mothers as well as increasing the nutritional content of the milk, treats acne, digestive tract issues, like obstructions in the pancreas, liver, gallbladder, and spleen, and detoxifies bloodstream.

Fennel

- **Precautions**: Not to be used in conjunction with tamoxifen, estrogen, contraceptives, or ciprofloxacin
- **Topical uses**: Essential oil can be used to treat muscle spasms of the respiratory, cardiovascular and digestive systems, useful for acne, and stomach cramps. Additionally, it is useful for the prevention of wound infection.
- **Used as teas**: Stimulates appetite, eases gas and bloating, and treats colic in infants, menstrual cramps, bronchitis, cough, and upper respiratory infections.

Ginger (*Zingiber Officinale*)

- **Precautions**: Not suitable for use when suffering from hyperacidity, peptic ulcers, or any hot inflammatory conditions. Not to be used in conjunction with blood-thinning drugs. A maximum of one gram is recommended for pregnant women.
- **Topical uses**: Footbaths for treating athlete's foot, gargle tea for treating sore throats, full-body baths for the treatment of sciatica, poor circulation, aching muscles, or chills. Compresses can be used to soothe symptoms of asthma when rested on the chest or back. When rested over the kidneys can alleviate pains due to kidney stones. Compresses can also be placed on over aching muscles, jaw for relief from toothache, or over joints to relieve arthritic pains.
- **Uses in teas**: Aids digestion, nausea, morning sickness, inflammation, circulation, and pain, promotes digestive secretions, and strengthens heart muscle tissue.

Licorice Root

- **Precautions**: May lead to vomiting, nausea, headaches, vertigo, increased blood pressure and heart rate, decreased potassium content, and fluid and sodium retention. It should not be used alongside diuretic drugs, hypotensive agents, digitoxin medicines, cardiac glycosides, steroids, monoamine oxidase inhibitors, or corticosteroids. It is also not for use during pregnancy.
- **Topical uses**: Mouthwash for the prevention of gingivitis, mouth sores, and tooth decay; hair wash for the treatment of dandruff and balding; use as a douche or lubrication for enemas and use to treat skin problems like eczema, psoriasis, itchy skin, wounds, inflamed eyelids, rashes, and dry eyes
- **Uses in teas**: Soothes abdominal issues like gas, colic, and bloating, improves pituitary functions, soothes irritated mucous membranes, used as a demulcent, emollient, and respiratory problems like coughs, bronchitis, and catarrh (mucus build-up in throat or nose).

Lemon Balm

- **Precautions**: Can reduce thyroid functions so it's not recommended for individuals with underactive thyroids
- **Topical uses**: Used in baths or as a compress for treating wounds, sunburn, boils, gout, insect bites, swelling, eczema, and tumors
- **Uses in teas**: Improves focus, treats chickenpox, herpes, colds, shingles, indigestion, flatulence, stomach problems, infant teething pains, soothes restlessness, depression, anxiety, and insomnia.

Marshmallow Root

- **Precaution**: This tea may affect the rate at which pharmaceuticals take effect.
- **Topical uses**: Wounds, baths, hemorrhoids, hair washes, mouthwash or gargle, varicose veins, burns, rectal irritation, sunburn, eye irritation, and vaginal dryness
- **Uses in teas**: Soothes inflammation of the urinary and digestive tract, promotes white cell production, cold infusions, soothes hyperactive immune systems, and soothes coughs and respiratory tract issues.

Nettle

- **Precautions**: Should be used under professional medical advice in people with yin deficiencies
- **Topical uses**: Baths for hemorrhoids, hair wash for balding and dandruff, compresses for treating wounds, sciatica, varicose veins, insect bites, heat rash, mastitis, tendonitis, gout, arthritis, chilblains, burns
- **Uses in teas**: Lowers blood sugar levels, stimulates healthy blood clotting, detoxifies, increases energy and limits appetite, relieves hemorrhage symptoms, supports general body health, improves mold and pollen resistance, reduces inflammation, and regulates mucous membrane functions.

Peppermint

Precautions: Nursing mothers can use it but, in moderation as excess amounts, can cause drying of the breast milk. Pregnant women should only have up to two cups a day. Not for people with gallstone problems, yin deficiency, and cold conditions.

- **Topical uses**: Used in baths for itchy skin and insect bites, mouthwash for the treatment of gingivitis and bad breath and soothes measles and chickenpox, steam inhalations for bronchitis, nasal congestion, asthma, nausea. It is also useful as a cold compress for headache and fever, and warm compress to treat lung infection, sinusitis, hives, backache, rheumatism, and joint inflammation.
- **Uses in teas**: Loosens phlegm, treats gas, colic in babies, muscle spasms, and stomach aches, possesses antiviral properties, and can be mixed with laxative concoctions in order to reduce the risk of gripe.

HERBS TO AVOID

Here is a list of 12 herbs that you may want to avoid or use with caution:

1. Comfrey: Comfrey has been linked to liver damage and should be avoided.
2. Sassafras: Sassafras contains safrole, which has been linked to cancer in animals and should be avoided.
3. Lobelia: Lobelia is a herb that can be toxic in high doses and should be used with caution.
4. Coltsfoot: Coltsfoot has been linked to liver damage and should be avoided.
5. Kava kava: Kava kava has been linked to liver damage and should be avoided.

6. Ephedra: Ephedra (also known as ma huang) has been linked to increased blood pressure and heart rate, and may increase the risk of heart attack and stroke.

7. Khat: Khat is a herb that contains cathinone, which has been linked to increased blood pressure and heart rate, and may increase the risk of heart attack and stroke.

8. Pennyroyal: Pennyroyal is a herb that has been linked to liver damage and may also have toxic effects on the heart.

9. Yohimbe: Yohimbe is a herb that has been linked to increased blood pressure and heart rate, and may increase the risk of heart attack and stroke.

10. Angelica: Angelica is a herb that has been linked to irregular heart rhythm and should be avoided by those with heart conditions.

11. Aconite: Aconite is a herb that has toxic effects on the heart and should be avoided.

12. Foxglove: Foxglove is a herb that has toxic effects on the heart and should be avoided.

In the next chapters we will take a look at our body's systems. They are important to understand, and although not the focus of this practical recipe book, it should help you as you consider what tea might help you

CHAPTER 4

Your Body Systems

The body's systems work together to maintain homeostasis, which is the state of steady internal, physical, and chemical conditions that the body needs to function. Each system plays a specific role in maintaining homeostasis and depends on the other systems to function properly. Here is a brief overview of how some of the body's systems work together:

- The circulatory system transports oxygen, nutrients, and hormones to cells and removes waste products. It works with the respiratory system to exchange oxygen and carbon dioxide.
- The digestive system breaks down food into nutrients that can be absorbed and used by the body. It works with the circulatory system to transport those nutrients to cells.
- The nervous system sends, receives, and processes sensory information. It works with the endocrine system to coordinate the body's responses to internal and

external stimuli.
- The musculoskeletal system allows the body to move and provides support and protection for internal organs. It works with the circulatory system to provide oxygen and nutrients to tissues and with the nervous system to coordinate movement.
- The immune system protects the body from infections and other diseases. It works with the circulatory system to transport immune cells and with the digestive system to eliminate pathogens.

This is just a small sample of the ways in which the body's systems work together. Every system in the body plays a vital role in maintaining homeostasis and overall health.

THE CIRCULATORY SYSTEM

The circulatory system, also known as the cardiovascular system, is a body system that is responsible for pumping and transporting blood, nutrients, oxygen, and hormones to and from cells. It is made up of the heart, blood vessels, and blood.

The main functions of the circulatory system include:

- Pumping blood: The heart is a muscular organ that pumps blood to the body's tissues and organs.
- Transporting oxygen and nutrients: Blood carries oxygen and nutrients from the lungs and digestive system to the body's cells.
- Removing waste products: Blood carries waste products, such as carbon dioxide and urea, away from the cells to be eliminated from the body.

- Regulating body temperature: Blood helps to regulate the body's temperature by carrying heat away from the body's core to the skin, where it can be dissipated.
- Protecting against infection: The circulatory system plays a role in the body's immune defense by carrying white blood cells and antibodies to areas of infection.

Overall, the circulatory system plays a vital role in maintaining the body's health by transporting oxygen, nutrients, and hormones to cells and removing waste products.

There are many herbs that are traditionally used to support the health and function of the circulatory system. Here are a few herbal tea recipes that you can try:

1. Hawthorn tea: Hawthorn is an herb that is traditionally used to support cardiovascular health and improve circulation. To make a cup of hawthorn tea, steep 1-2 teaspoons of dried hawthorn berries or leaves in a cup of hot water for 5-10 minutes.
2. Cayenne pepper tea: Cayenne pepper is a spicy herb that is traditionally used to improve circulation and support cardiovascular health. To make a cup of cayenne pepper tea, steep 1-2 teaspoons of dried cayenne pepper in a cup of hot water for 5-10 minutes.
3. Ginkgo biloba tea: Ginkgo biloba is an herb that is traditionally used to improve circulation and support cognitive function. To make a cup of ginkgo biloba tea, steep 1-2 teaspoons of dried ginkgo biloba leaves in a cup of hot water for 5-10 minutes.
4. Horse chestnut tea: Horse chestnut is an herb that is traditionally used to improve circulation and reduce inflammation. To make a cup of horse chestnut tea,

steep 1-2 teaspoons of dried horse chestnut seeds or leaves in a cup of hot water for 5-10 minutes.

5. Dandelion tea: Dandelion is an herb that is traditionally used to support liver health and improve circulation. To make a cup of dandelion tea, steep 1-2 teaspoons of dried dandelion leaves in a cup of hot water for 5-10 minutes.

As a simple example of how to work with this information, one area of interest is how certain herbs can help increase oxygen in the blood, which can help to reduce the appearance of dark circles and eye bags, and potentially reduce the risk of bruising.

The skin around the eyes is thin and delicate, and it is not uncommon for people to develop dark circles and eye bags as they age. Dark circles can be caused by a number of factors, including genetics, lack of sleep, and poor nutrition. However, a lack of oxygen in the blood can also contribute to the appearance of dark circles. When the skin around the eyes is not getting enough oxygen, it can appear darker and more tired.

Herbs can be a powerful tool for increasing oxygen in the blood and helping to reduce the appearance of dark circles. Some of the most commonly used herbs for this purpose include ginkgo biloba, hawthorn (mentioned above), and gotu kola. These herbs work by improving circulation and increasing blood flow, which in turn helps to deliver more oxygen to the skin around the eyes.

Ginkgo biloba is a well-known herb that has been used for centuries to improve circulation and increase oxygen in the blood. It is believed to work by dilating blood vessels, which allows for better blood flow and increased oxygen delivery to the skin. Ginkgo biloba is also rich in antioxidants, which can help to protect the skin from damage caused by free radicals.

Hawthorn works by improving circulation and strengthening

the walls of blood vessels, which in turn helps to improve the delivery of oxygen to the skin. Hawthorn is also believed to have a mild sedative effect, which can help to reduce stress and improve sleep, both of which can contribute to the appearance of dark circles.

Gotu kola is another herb that has been used for centuries to improve circulation and increase oxygen in the blood. It is believed to work by improving the elasticity of blood vessels, which in turn helps to improve blood flow and increase the delivery of oxygen to the skin. gotu kola is also rich in antioxidants, which can help to protect the skin from damage caused by free radicals.

Herbal teas made from these herbs can be a simple and effective way to help increase oxygen in the blood and reduce the appearance of dark circles. To make a tea, simply add one or two teaspoons of dried herbs to a cup of boiling water. Let the tea steep for five to 10 minutes, then strain and drink. It is recommended to drink two to three cups of herbal tea per day to see the best results.

In addition to helping reduce the appearance of dark circles, increasing oxygen in the blood may also help to reduce the risk of bruising. Bruising occurs when blood vessels are damaged and blood leaks into the surrounding tissue, causing a discoloration of the skin. A lack of oxygen in the blood can contribute to the formation of bruises, as it makes blood vessels more fragile and prone to breaking. By increasing the oxygen levels in the blood, herbs can help to improve the health and strength of blood vessels, reducing the risk of bruising.

THE DIGESTIVE SYSTEM

The digestive system is a group of organs that work together to convert food into energy and nutrients that the body needs to function. The main functions of the digestive system include:

- Ingestion: The process of eating and swallowing food.
- Digestion: The process of breaking down food into smaller molecules that can be absorbed and used by the body. Digestion begins in the mouth with chewing and is completed in the small intestine with the help of enzymes produced by the pancreas, liver, and small intestine.
- Absorption: The process of taking in nutrients from food and drink into the body. Nutrients are absorbed from the small intestine into the bloodstream and transported to the liver for processing and storage.
- Elimination: The process of removing waste products from the body. The large intestine absorbs water and electrolytes from the remaining indigestible food matter, and the rectum and anus eliminate the solid waste products from the body.

Overall, the digestive system plays a vital role in maintaining the body's health by converting food into energy and nutrients and eliminating waste products.

Here are a few herbal tea recipes that may support digestive system health:

1. Chamomile tea: Chamomile is a calming herb that has been traditionally used to help with sleep and relaxation. It has also been used to help with digestive issues. To make chamomile tea, steep 1-2 teaspoons of dried chamomile flowers in 8 ounces of hot water for 5-10 minutes.
2. Ginger tea: Ginger is a warming herb that has been traditionally used to help with nausea and inflammation. It has also been used to help with

digestive issues. To make ginger tea, steep 1-2 teaspoons of sliced fresh ginger or 1 teaspoon of dried ginger powder in 8 ounces of hot water for 5-10 minutes.

3. Peppermint tea: Peppermint is a refreshing herb that has been traditionally used to help with digestion and headaches. To make peppermint tea, steep 1-2 teaspoons of dried peppermint leaves in 8 ounces of hot water for 5-10 minutes.

4. Fennel tea: Fennel is an herb that has been traditionally used to help with digestion and bloating. To make fennel tea, steep 1-2 teaspoons of dried fennel seeds in 8 ounces of hot water for 5-10 minutes.

5. Licorice tea: Licorice is an herb that has been traditionally used to help with digestive issues and to soothe the throat. To make licorice tea, steep 1-2 teaspoons of dried licorice root in 8 ounces of hot water for 5-10 minutes.

THE ENDOCRINE SYSTEM

The endocrine system is a network of glands that produce and secrete hormones, chemical messengers that help regulate the body's functions. The endocrine system plays a vital role in maintaining homeostasis, which is the state of steady internal, physical, and chemical conditions that the body needs to function.

The main functions of the endocrine system include:

- Regulating metabolism: Hormones produced by the endocrine system help regulate the body's metabolism, which is the process of converting food into energy.

- Controlling growth and development: Hormones produced by the endocrine system help control growth and development during childhood and adolescence.
- Regulating mood and behavior: Hormones produced by the endocrine system, such as serotonin and cortisol, can affect mood and behavior.
- Regulating reproduction: Hormones produced by the endocrine system, such as testosterone and estrogen, play a role in regulating the reproductive system.

The endocrine system is especially important for women and women's health and, like all body systems there are many herbs that are used to support its health and function. Here are just a few herbal tea recipes to try:

1. Ashwagandha tea: Ashwagandha is an herb that is traditionally used to support the endocrine system and help the body cope with stress. To make a cup of ashwagandha tea, steep 1-2 teaspoons of dried ashwagandha root in a cup of hot water for 5-10 minutes.
2. Maca tea: Maca is an herb that is traditionally used to support hormonal balance and improve energy levels. To make a cup of maca tea, steep 1-2 teaspoons of dried maca root in a cup of hot water for 5-10 minutes.
3. Holy basil tea: Holy basil is an herb that is traditionally used to reduce stress and support the endocrine system. To make a cup of holy basil tea, steep 1-2 teaspoons of dried holy basil leaves in a cup of hot water for 5-10 minutes.
4. Licorice root tea: Licorice root is an herb that is traditionally used to support the endocrine system and

help the body cope with stress. To make a cup of licorice root tea, steep 1-2 teaspoons of dried licorice root in a cup of hot water for 5-10 minutes.

5. Rhodiola tea: Rhodiola is an herb that is traditionally used to improve energy levels and support the endocrine system. To make a cup of rhodiola tea, steep 1-2 teaspoons of dried rhodiola root in a cup of hot water for 5-10 minutes. Rhodiola is sometimes referred to as "golden root" or "arctic root" due to its golden-yellow color and its ability to thrive in cold, high-altitude environments. Some people also use rhodiola as a natural supplement to improve physical and mental performance, and to reduce stress and fatigue.

THE IMMUNE SYSTEM

The immune system is a complex network of organs, tissues, and cells that work together to defend the body against infection and disease. The main functions of the immune system include:

- Identifying and eliminating foreign substances: The immune system is able to recognize and eliminate foreign substances, such as bacteria, viruses, and toxins, that can cause illness or infection.
- Protecting against infection: The immune system produces white blood cells and antibodies that help protect the body against infection and disease.
- Remembering past infections: The immune system is able to "remember" past infections and quickly respond to them if they occur again. This is how vaccines work – they expose the body to a small, harmless amount of a

virus or bacteria, which allows the immune system to create immunity to that particular disease.

- Maintaining the body's overall health: The immune system helps to maintain the body's overall health by attacking and eliminating foreign substances that can cause illness or infection.

Overall, the immune system plays a vital role in protecting the body against infection and disease

Here are a some herbal tea recipes that may support your immune system:

1. Echinacea tea: Echinacea is an herb that has been traditionally used to help with the common cold and other respiratory infections. It has also been used to support immune system health. To make echinacea tea, steep 1-2 teaspoons of dried echinacea root or flowers in 8 ounces of hot water for 5-10 minutes.

2. Astragalus tea: Astragalus is an herb that has been traditionally used to support immune system health. To make astragalus tea, steep 1-2 teaspoons of dried astragalus root in 8 ounces of hot water for 5-10 minutes.

3. Ginger tea: Ginger is a warming herb that has been traditionally used to help with nausea and inflammation. It has also been used to support immune system health. To make ginger tea, steep 1-2 teaspoons of sliced fresh ginger or 1 teaspoon of dried ginger powder in 8 ounces of hot water for 5-10 minutes.

4. Turmeric tea: Turmeric is a potent antioxidant that has been traditionally used to help with inflammation and pain. It has also been used to support immune system

health. To make turmeric tea, steep 1 teaspoon of turmeric powder in 8 ounces of hot water for 5-10 minutes. You can also add a pinch of black pepper to help increase the absorption of the turmeric.

5. Reishi mushroom tea: Reishi mushroom is an herb that has been traditionally used to support immune system health. To make reishi mushroom tea, steep 1-2 teaspoons of dried reishi mushroom in 8 ounces of hot water for 5-10 minutes.

THE LYMPHATIC SYSTEM

The lymphatic system is a part of the immune system and is responsible for the production, maintenance, and circulation of lymph, a clear fluid that helps to protect the body against infection and disease. The lymphatic system is made up of a network of lymph vessels, lymph nodes, and organs, such as the spleen and thymus.

The main functions of the lymphatic system include:

- Filtering lymph fluid: Lymph vessels filter lymph fluid as it flows through the body, removing waste products, bacteria, and other substances.
- Transporting immune cells: Lymph vessels transport immune cells, such as lymphocytes and monocytes, throughout the body to help protect against infection and disease.
- Storing immune cells: Lymph nodes, which are small, bean-shaped structures located throughout the body, store immune cells and produce more immune cells when needed.

- Absorbing excess fluid: The lymphatic system helps to drain excess fluid from tissues and return it to the circulatory system.

Overall, the lymphatic system plays a vital role in maintaining the body's immune defenses and supporting the health of tissues and organs.

Here are a a selection of herbal tea recipes that may support lymphatic system health:

1. Red clover tea: Red clover is an herb that has been traditionally used to help with menopausal symptoms and as a natural expectorant. It has also been used to support lymphatic system health. To make red clover tea, steep 1-2 teaspoons of dried red clover flowers in 8 ounces of hot water for 5-10 minutes.

2. Echinacea tea: Echinacea is an herb that has been traditionally used to help with the common cold and other respiratory infections. It has also been used to support lymphatic system health. To make echinacea tea, steep 1-2 teaspoons of dried echinacea root or flowers in 8 ounces of hot water for 5-10 minutes.

3. Calendula tea: Calendula is an herb that has been traditionally used to help with skin irritation and inflammation. It has also been used to support lymphatic system health. To make calendula tea, steep 1-2 teaspoons of dried calendula flowers in 8 ounces of hot water for 5-10 minutes.

4. Cleavers tea: Cleavers is an herb that has been traditionally used to support lymphatic system health. To make cleavers tea, steep 1-2 teaspoons of dried cleavers in 8 ounces of hot water for 5-10 minutes.

5. Goldenseal tea: Goldenseal is an herb that has been traditionally used to support immune system health. It has also been used to support lymphatic system health. To make goldenseal tea, steep 1-2 teaspoons of dried goldenseal root in 8 ounces of hot water for 5-10 minutes.

THE MUSCULOSKELETAL SYSTEM

Once more, here are a few herbal tea recipes that may support musculoskeletal health:

1. Turmeric tea: Turmeric is a potent antioxidant that has been traditionally used to help with inflammation and pain. To make turmeric tea, steep 1 teaspoon of turmeric powder in 8 ounces of hot water for 5-10 minutes. You can also add a pinch of black pepper to help increase the absorption of the turmeric.
2. Ginger tea: Ginger is a warming herb that has been traditionally used to help with nausea and inflammation. To make ginger tea, steep 1-2 teaspoons of sliced fresh ginger or 1 teaspoon of dried ginger powder in 8 ounces of hot water for 5-10 minutes.
3. White willow bark tea: White willow bark is an herb that has been traditionally used to help with pain and inflammation. To make white willow bark tea, steep 1-2 teaspoons of dried white willow bark in 8 ounces of hot water for 5-10 minutes.
4. Devils claw tea: Devil's claw is an herb that has been traditionally used to help with pain and inflammation. To make devil's claw tea, steep 1-2 teaspoons of dried

devil's claw root in 8 ounces of hot water for 5-10 minutes.

5. Marjoram tea: Marjoram is an herb that has been traditionally used to help with digestion and to reduce muscle spasms. To make marjoram tea, steep 1-2 teaspoons of dried marjoram in 8 ounces of hot water for 5-10 minutes.

It's important to note that these are just a few examples and that other herbs, such as boswellia and bromelain, may also support musculoskeletal health. It's always a good idea to consult with a healthcare professional before consuming any herbs, especially if you have a medical condition or are taking medications.

THE NERVOUS SYSTEM

There are many herbs that are traditionally used to support the health and function of the nervous system. For example:

1. Chamomile tea: Chamomile is a soothing herb that is traditionally used to reduce anxiety and promote relaxation. To make a cup of chamomile tea, steep 1-2 teaspoons of dried chamomile flowers in a cup of hot water for 5-10 minutes.
2. Lemon balm tea: Lemon balm is a calming herb that is often used to reduce stress and improve sleep. To make a cup of lemon balm tea, steep 1-2 teaspoons of dried lemon balm leaves in a cup of hot water for 5-10 minutes.
3. Passionflower tea: Passionflower is a herb that is traditionally used to help with anxiety and sleep. To make a cup of passionflower tea, steep 1-2 teaspoons of

dried passionflower in a cup of hot water for 5-10 minutes.

4. Peppermint tea: Peppermint is a refreshing herb that is traditionally used to improve digestion and reduce stress. To make a cup of peppermint tea, steep 1-2 teaspoons of dried peppermint leaves in a cup of hot water for 5-10 minutes.

5. Valerian root tea: Valerian root is an herb that is traditionally used to promote relaxation and improve sleep. To make a cup of valerian root tea, steep 1-2 teaspoons of dried valerian root in a cup of hot water for 5-10 minutes.

THE RESPIRATORY SYSTEM

Here are a few herbal tea recipes that may support respiratory system health:

1. Echinacea tea: Echinacea is an herb that has been traditionally used to help with the common cold and other respiratory infections. To make echinacea tea, steep 1-2 teaspoons of dried echinacea root or flowers in 8 ounces of hot water for 5-10 minutes.

2. Thyme tea: Thyme is an herb that has been traditionally used to help with respiratory issues and as a natural expectorant. To make thyme tea, steep 1-2 teaspoons of dried thyme leaves in 8 ounces of hot water for 5-10 minutes.

3. Mullein tea: Mullein is an herb that has been traditionally used to help with respiratory issues and as a natural expectorant. To make mullein tea, steep 1-2

teaspoons of dried mullein leaves in 8 ounces of hot water for 5-10 minutes.

4. Peppermint tea: Peppermint is a refreshing herb that has been traditionally used to help with digestion and headaches. It has also been used to help with respiratory issues. To make peppermint tea, steep 1-2 teaspoons of dried peppermint leaves in 8 ounces of hot water for 5-10 minutes.

5. Licorice tea: Licorice is an herb that has been traditionally used to help with digestive issues and to soothe the throat. To make licorice tea, steep 1-2 teaspoons of dried licorice root in 8 ounces of hot water for 5-10 minutes.

If you have a specific problem or are trying to work with a particular organ it is always better to do some research - below are just two examples of the types of herbs that can work with two organs that tend to raise the most questions. In this case always consult with a professional before consuming any herbs by any method.

LIVER

Here are a few herbal tea recipes that may support liver health:

- Dandelion tea: Dandelion is a liver-supporting herb that has been traditionally used to help with digestion and as a natural diuretic. To make dandelion tea, steep 1-2 teaspoons of dried dandelion leaves in 8 ounces of hot water for 5-10 minutes.
- Milk thistle tea: Milk thistle is an herb that has been traditionally used to support liver health. To make milk thistle tea, steep 1-2 teaspoons of dried milk thistle seeds in 8 ounces of hot water for 5-10 minutes.
- Turmeric tea: Turmeric is a potent antioxidant that has been traditionally used to help with inflammation and pain. To make turmeric tea, steep 1 teaspoon of turmeric powder in 8 ounces of hot water for 5-10 minutes. You can also add a pinch of black pepper to help increase the absorption of the turmeric.
- Lemon balm tea: Lemon balm is an herb that has been traditionally used to help with sleep and to reduce anxiety. To make lemon balm tea, steep 1-2 teaspoons of dried lemon balm leaves in 8 ounces of hot water for 5-10 minutes.
- Peppermint tea: Peppermint is a refreshing herb that has been traditionally used to help with digestion and headaches. To make peppermint tea, steep 1-2 teaspoons of dried peppermint leaves in 8 ounces of hot water for 5-10 minutes.

KIDNEY

Here are a few herbal tea recipes that may support kidney health:

1. Dandelion tea: Dandelion is an herb that has been traditionally used to help with digestion and as a natural diuretic. To make dandelion tea, steep 1-2 teaspoons of dried dandelion leaves in 8 ounces of hot water for 5-10 minutes.
2. Nettle tea: Nettle is an herb that has been traditionally used to help with allergy symptoms and as a natural diuretic. To make nettle tea, steep 1-2 teaspoons of dried nettle leaves in 8 ounces of hot water for 5-10 minutes.
3. Green tea: Green tea is an herbal tea that is high in antioxidants and has been traditionally used to support overall health. To make green tea, steep 1 teaspoon of green tea leaves in 8 ounces of hot water for 2-3 minutes.
4. Lemon balm tea: Lemon balm is an herb that has been traditionally used to help with sleep and to reduce anxiety. To make lemon balm tea, steep 1-2 teaspoons of dried lemon balm leaves in 8 ounces of hot water for 5-10 minutes.
5. Parsley tea: Parsley is an herb that has been traditionally used as a natural diuretic. To make parsley tea, steep 1-2 teaspoons of dried parsley leaves in 8 ounces of hot water for 5-10 minutes.

CHAPTER 5
Herbs and Teas for common problems

In the following pages we will list tea recipes for many of the most common problems.

You will notice that each tea recipe is very similar (and covered in a previous chapter). They are included for each tea in here, so that you know what to do for each tea and so that you can use this book as a grab-and-go.

Also, and as has been mentioned, you will want to vary the steeping time depending on whether you are using fresh herbs or dried herbs. Fresh herbs include the flowers, seeds, leaves or bark (longer for bark and less time for flowers).

In almost all cases they are made as follows:

- 1 cup water (8 oz)
- 1-2 teaspoons dried herb (no less than 2 of the fresh herb)
- Honey or lemon (optional)

Instructions:

- Boil the water in a kettle or on the stove.
- Place the herb in a mug.
- Pour the hot water over the herb and let it steep for 5-10 minutes
- Remove the leaves from the mug.
- Add honey or lemon to taste (or other flavor choice - see below), if desired.

Some herbs can be used for different problems and they are included for each problem where they are relevant.

The intention is to make this book as easy as possible and to highlight just how simple it is to make herbal teas a part of your day-to-day life.

Once again, it's important to note that these teas may not be a cure your problem and that results may vary from person to person. You should always consult with a healthcare professional if you have concerns about your health or if you are taking other medications.

Before we begin it is useful to know what you can add to improve the taste of your tea.

There are many ways to make herbal tea taste better, and the best method will depend on your personal preferences. Here are a few common additives that people use to make herbal tea taste better:

- Honey: Honey is a sweetener that can add a touch of sweetness to herbal tea. It's also a natural cough suppressant, so it can be especially helpful in soothing sore throats.
- Lemon: Lemon is a citrus fruit that can add a bright, refreshing flavor to herbal tea. It's also rich in vitamin C, which may help to support immune system health.
- Mint: Mint is a refreshing herb that can add a cool, invigorating flavor to herbal tea. It's also been traditionally used to help with digestion.
- Ginger: Ginger is a warming herb that can add a spicy, zesty flavor to herbal tea. It's also been traditionally used to help with nausea and inflammation.
- Cinnamon: Cinnamon is a spice that can add a sweet, warm flavor to herbal tea. It's also been traditionally used to help with digestion and to regulate blood sugar levels.

The most common flavor mix is honey and lemon but this taste won't work for all teas and tastes. I have added this to some of the recipes for guidance.

You can also add your herbs to green tea - There are several herbs that go well with green tea for health benefits. Some options include:

1. Mint: Mint has a refreshing flavor and can help with digestion.
2. Lemon balm: Lemon balm has a citrusy flavor and is believed to have calming effects.
3. Basil: Basil has a sweet, slightly spicy flavor and is thought to have anti-inflammatory properties.

4. Ginger: Ginger has a spicy, warming flavor and is believed to have anti-inflammatory and immune-boosting effects.

5. Fennel: Fennel has a licorice-like flavor and is believed to have digestive and diuretic properties.

In the following page we list the most common ailments and easy-to-prepare herbal teas that may help.

ACID REFLUX

Acid reflux, also known as gastroesophageal reflux disease (GERD), is a condition where stomach acid flows back up into the esophagus, causing discomfort and a burning sensation in the chest and throat and can lead to heartburn, regurgitation, and other symptoms. It is estimated that up to 20% of the population experiences acid reflux symptoms at least once a week.

Although there are over-the-counter medicines available, many people turn to herbal teas as a natural remedy. Here, we will explore some of the most effective herbal teas for acid reflux, as well as the reasons why they are effective, and what causes acid reflux in the first place.

One of the most popular herbs is **Chamomile**. Its calming and soothing properties makes it an ideal choice as it can help to soothe the burning sensations and reduce inflammation in the esophagus. Chamomile also has natural antispasmodic properties, which can help to relax the muscles in the digestive tract and relieve any spasms that may be contributing to acid reflux.

Ginger is well known for its ability to calm the digestive system and reduce symptoms of acid reflux. This is due in part to its natural anti-inflammatory properties, as well as its ability to reduce nausea and promote healthy digestion. Ginger also contains compounds that help to neutralize stomach acid, which can help to prevent acid reflux from occurring in the first place. Some people find that drinking a cup of ginger tea before meals can help to prevent acid reflux, while others may find relief by drinking ginger tea throughout the day as needed.

Peppermint is another herb that is commonly used to help with acid reflux but it is not the best. Peppermint has natural antispasmodic properties that can help to soothe the digestive tract and reduce the frequency of the condition. This is because peppermint has the ability to relax the muscles in the digestive tract, reducing the pressure on the esophageal sphincter and preventing stomach acid from flowing back into the esophagus. However peppermint tea can relax the lower esophageal sphincter too effectively and cause acid to flow back into the esophagus. In this case, drinking chamomile tea or licorice root tea might be a better choice.

Licorice root is believed to help soothe the digestive system and reduce symptoms of acid reflux by promoting healthy digestion and reducing inflammation in the digestive tract.

Like Ginger, licorice root also contains natural compounds that have been shown to help neutralize stomach acid. You can opt to drink licorice root tea before meals or throughout the day as needed.

You can also try Marshmallow root or slippery elm tea.

While these herbs are generally considered effective, it's important to keep in mind that not all herbs are right for everyone and that hat while these herbal teas can be helpful for digestive problems, they are not a cure-all.

When it comes to acid reflux, it's also important to consider the underlying causes. There are many different factors that can contribute to the problem, including diet, lifestyle, and genetics and understanding these triggers can help manage your symptoms. Other than medical conditions such as hiatal hernias or gastroesophage the most common day-to-day triggers are outlined below.

Certain foods can trigger acid reflux by relaxing the lower esophageal sphincter (LES), which allows acid to flow back into the esophagus.

- Chocolate including chocolate milk and cocoa contain a substance called methylxanthine, which can relax the lower esophageal sphincter (LES).
- Alcohol and the caffeine in coffee and tea also relaxes the LES.

- Fatty or dried foods can slow digestions and delay the opening of the LES.
- Citrus fruits like oranges, lemons and limes along with spicy foods, alcohol, tomatoes and tomato-based products all irritate the esophagus triggering reflux symptoms.
- Garlic and onions contain sulfurous compounds that can trigger symptoms
- Carbonated drinks can increase pressure in the stomach and force acid into the esophagus.

In addition to food and drink triggers, there are also certain lifestyle factors that can trigger acid reflux. For example:

- Eating large meals can put pressure on the LES and eating close to bedtime can increase the risk (when you lie down it is easier for acid to flow back into the esophagus).
- Wearing tight clothing or being overweight can put pressure on the LES triggering symptoms while smoking and stress relaxes the LES.

ACNE

Acne is a common skin condition that affects millions of people. It is characterized by the appearance of pimples, blackheads, and whiteheads on the face, neck, back, and chest. Acne is caused by a complex interplay of factors, including hormonal changes, genetics, bacteria, and lifestyle habits.

Hormonal changes play a crucial role in the development of acne. During puberty, androgen hormone levels increase, leading to the production of more oil (sebum) by the sebaceous glands. This can clog the pores and create an ideal environment for the growth of the bacteria Propionibacterium acnes, which can trigger inflammation and result in acne breakouts.

Genetics can also play a role in acne susceptibility, as the condition tends to run in families. Certain genetic variations may affect the way the body responds to hormonal changes and how susceptible the skin is to developing acne.

Lifestyle factors, such as diet, stress, and skin care habits, can also contribute to breakouts while a diet high in sugar and processed foods can trigger inflammation and exacerbate symptoms.

Stress can also be a trigger by causing hormonal imbalances and increasing sebum production and using products that are too harsh or not appropriate for your skin type can irritate the skin and trigger a breakout.

Herbs have been used for centuries to treat acne and its symptoms. Some of the most commonly used herbs for acne include:

- Tea tree oil: This essential oil has antimicrobial and anti-inflammatory properties. It is often used topically to treat pimples and other acne-related skin problems.
- Green tea contains antioxidants and anti-inflammatory compounds that can help reduce the redness and swelling associated with acne. It can be applied topically to the skin or consumed as a tea (see below).
- Aloe vera has anti-inflammatory and moisturizing properties that make it an effective herb for treating acne. It can be applied topically to help soothe and hydrate the skin.
- Witch hazel is an astringent that helps to tighten and tone the skin. Applied topically to the skin it helps to reduce inflammation.

- Turmeric contains anti-inflammatory compounds that can help reduce the redness and swelling associated with acne. It can be applied topically to the skin or consumed as a supplement to help soothe acne-prone skin.

Other teas include Dandelion - its diuretic properties and may help to flush toxins from the body - and Lemon Balm with antiviral and antibacterial properties which may help to reduce inflammation.

One of the best herbs that has been proven to help with acne caused by puberty is green tea.

Green tea is rich in antioxidants and anti-inflammatory compounds, such as epicatechin, gallate, and catechins, which have been shown to help reduce the redness and swelling associated with acne. In a study published in the Journal of Drugs in Dermatology, green tea was found to be effective in reducing the number of pimples and improving overall skin clarity in individuals with acne-prone skin

Another study published in the International Journal of Dermatology found that topical application of green tea extract reduced the number of pimples and improved skin texture in patients with moderate to severe acne.

In addition to its anti-inflammatory properties, green tea has antimicrobial effects that help to fight the bacteria Propionibacterium acnes, which is a major contributor to acne breakouts. Drinking green tea or applying it topically to the skin can help soothe acne-prone skin and reduce the appearance of pimples.

However, it is important to note that green tea is not appropriate for everyone and may not be safe for individuals with certain medical conditions. For example, green tea can interact with blood thinners and can increase the risk of bleeding in individuals taking these medications. Additionally, green tea may cause skin irritation in some individuals, particularly those with sensitive skin.

ANXIETY

There are many causes of anxiety but one of the underlying causes is often stress. The best teas will help your relax, or sleep (or both), two of the best remedies for anxiety.

Here are a few herbal tea recipes that may help with anxiety:

1. Lemon balm tea: Lemon balm is an herb that has been traditionally used to help with anxiety and to improve sleep.
2. Chamomile tea: Chamomile is a calming herb that has been traditionally used to help with sleep and relaxation. It has also been used to help with anxiety. Lavender tea: Lavender is an herb that has been traditionally used to help with relaxation and to improve sleep. It has also been used to help with anxiety. To make lavender tea, steep 1-2 teaspoons of dried lavender flowers (no less than two if you are using fresh lavender) in 8 ounces of hot water for 5-10 minutes.
3. Valerian root tea: Valerian root is an herb that has been traditionally used to help with anxiety and to improve sleep. To make valerian root tea, steep 1-2 teaspoons of dried valerian root in 8 ounces of hot water for 5-10 minutes.
4. Peppermint tea: Peppermint is a refreshing herb that has been traditionally used to help with digestion and headaches. It has also been used to help with anxiety. To make peppermint tea, steep 1-2 teaspoons of dried

peppermint leaves in 8 ounces of hot water for 5-10 minutes.

ARTHRITIS

One of the causes of Arthritis is inflammation. It is a common condition that often comes with age and is also influenced by the hormonal changes in women during menopause.

Here are a few herbal tea recipes that may help:

1. Ginger tea: Ginger is a herb that has natural anti-inflammatory properties and may help to reduce symptoms of arthritis. To make ginger tea, steep one teaspoon of freshly grated ginger in one cup of boiling water for 5-10 minutes. Strain and drink one cup of the tea several times per day
2. Turmeric tea: Turmeric is a herb that has natural anti-inflammatory properties and may help to reduce symptoms of arthritis. To make turmeric tea, steep one teaspoon of turmeric powder in one cup of boiling water for 5-10 minutes. Strain and drink one cup of the tea several times per day.
3. Black pepper tea: Black pepper is a herb that has natural anti-inflammatory properties and may help to reduce symptoms of arthritis. To make black pepper tea, steep one teaspoon of black peppercorns in one cup of boiling water for 5-10 minutes. Strain and drink one cup of the tea several times per day.
4. Boswellia tea: Boswellia is a herb that has natural anti-inflammatory properties and may help to reduce symptoms of arthritis. To make boswellia tea, steep one teaspoon of dried boswellia resin in one cup of boiling

water for 5-10 minutes. Strain and drink one cup of the tea several times per day.

ASTHMA

1. Licorice tea: Licorice is an herb that has been traditionally used to help with digestive issues and to soothe the throat. It has also been used to help with asthma. To make licorice tea, steep 1-2 teaspoons of dried licorice root in 8 ounces of hot water for 5-10 minutes.

2. Mullein tea: Mullein is an herb that has been traditionally used to help with respiratory issues and to soothe the throat. It has also been used to help with asthma. To make mullein tea, steep 1-2 teaspoons of dried mullein leaves in 8 ounces of hot water for 5-10 minutes.

3. Eucalyptus tea: Eucalyptus is an herb that has been traditionally used to help with respiratory issues and to soothe the throat. It has also been used to help with asthma. To make eucalyptus tea, steep 1-2 teaspoons of dried eucalyptus leaves in 8 ounces of hot water for 5-10 minutes.

4. Thyme tea: Thyme is an herb that has been traditionally used to help with respiratory issues and to soothe the throat. It has also been used to help with asthma. To make thyme tea, steep 1-2 teaspoons of dried thyme leaves in 8 ounces of hot water for 5-10 minutes.

5. Ginger tea: Ginger is a warming herb that has been traditionally used to help with nausea and inflammation. It has also been used to help with asthma.

To make ginger tea, steep 1-2 teaspoons of sliced fresh ginger or 1 teaspoon of dried ginger powder in 8 ounces of hot water for 5-10 minutes

BRONCHITIS AND LARYNGITIS

Here are a few herbal tea recipes that may help with bronchitis:

1. Licorice tea: Licorice is an herb that has been traditionally used to help with digestive issues and to soothe the throat. It has also been used to help with bronchitis and laryngitis. To make licorice tea, steep 1-2 teaspoons of dried licorice root in 8 ounces of hot water for 5-10 minutes.
2. Mullein tea: Mullein is an herb that has been traditionally used to help with respiratory issues and to soothe the throat. It has also been used to help with bronchitis and laryngitis. To make mullein tea, steep 1-2 teaspoons of dried mullein leaves in 8 ounces of hot water for 5-10 minutes.
3. Eucalyptus tea: Eucalyptus is an herb that has been traditionally used to help with respiratory issues and to soothe the throat. It has also been used to help with bronchitis and laryngitis. To make eucalyptus tea, steep 1-2 teaspoons of dried eucalyptus leaves in 8 ounces of hot water for 5-10 minutes.
4. Thyme tea: Thyme is an herb that has been traditionally used to help with respiratory issues and to soothe the throat. It has also been used to help with bronchitis and laryngitis. To make thyme tea, steep 1-2 teaspoons of dried thyme leaves in 8 ounces of hot water for 5-10 minutes.

5. Ginger tea: Ginger is a warming herb that has been traditionally used to help with nausea and inflammation. It has also been used to help with bronchitis and laryngitis. To make ginger tea, steep 1-2 teaspoons of sliced fresh ginger or 1 teaspoon of dried ginger powder in 8 ounces of hot water for 5-10 minutes.

CHEST CONGESTION

Here are a few herbal tea recipes that may help to loosen congestion in the chest:

1. Peppermint tea: Peppermint is a herb that has natural decongestant and expectorant properties and may help to loosen congestion in the chest. To make peppermint tea, steep one teaspoon of dried peppermint leaves in one cup of boiling water for 5-10 minutes. Strain and drink one cup of the tea several times per day.

2. Eucalyptus tea: Eucalyptus is a herb that has natural decongestant and expectorant properties and may help to loosen congestion in the chest. To make eucalyptus tea, steep one teaspoon of dried eucalyptus leaves in one cup of boiling water for 5-10 minutes. Strain and drink one cup of the tea several times per day.

3. Thyme tea: Thyme is a herb that has natural expectorant properties and may help to loosen congestion in the chest. To make thyme tea, steep one teaspoon of dried thyme leaves in one cup of boiling water for 5-10 minutes. Strain and drink one cup of the tea several times per day.

4. Licorice root tea: Licorice root is a herb that is believed to have expectorant properties and may help to loosen congestion in the chest. To make licorice root tea, steep one teaspoon of dried licorice root in one cup of boiling water for 5-10 minutes. Strain and drink one cup of the tea several times per day.

CONSTIPATION

1. Senna tea: Senna is a herb that has a natural laxative effect and may help to relieve constipation. To make senna tea, steep one teaspoon of dried senna leaves in one cup of boiling water for 5-10 minutes. Strain and drink one cup of the tea per day.
2. Dandelion tea: Dandelion is a herb that has a natural diuretic effect and may help to relieve constipation. To make dandelion tea, steep one teaspoon of dried dandelion leaves in one cup of boiling water for 5-10 minutes. Strain and drink one cup of the tea per day.
3. Cascara tea: Cascara is a herb that has a natural laxative effect and may help to relieve constipation. To make cascara tea, steep one teaspoon of dried cascara bark in one cup of boiling water for 5-10 minutes. Strain and drink one cup of the tea per day.
4. Fennel tea: Fennel is a herb that has been shown to improve digestion and may help to relieve constipation. To make fennel tea, steep one teaspoon of dried fennel seeds in one cup of boiling water for 5-10 minutes. Strain and drink one cup of the tea per day.

COPD

Here are a few herbal tea recipes that may help with COPD (chronic obstructive pulmonary disease):

1. Licorice tea: Licorice is an herb that has been traditionally used to help with respiratory issues and to soothe the throat. It has also been used to help with COPD. To make licorice tea, steep 1-2 teaspoons of dried licorice root in 8 ounces of hot water for 5-10 minutes.

2. Mullein tea: Mullein is an herb that has been traditionally used to help with respiratory issues and to soothe the throat. It has also been used to help with COPD. To make mullein tea, steep 1-2 teaspoons of dried mullein leaves in 8 ounces of hot water for 5-10 minutes.

3. Eucalyptus tea: Eucalyptus is an herb that has been traditionally used to help with respiratory issues and to soothe the throat. It has also been used to help with COPD. To make eucalyptus tea, steep 1-2 teaspoons of dried eucalyptus leaves in 8 ounces of hot water for 5-10 minutes.

4. Thyme tea: Thyme is an herb that has been traditionally used to help with respiratory issues and to soothe the throat. It has also been used to help with COPD. To make thyme tea, steep 1-2 teaspoons of dried thyme leaves in 8 ounces of hot water for 5-10 minutes.

5. Ginger tea: Ginger is a warming herb that has been traditionally used to help with nausea and inflammation. It has also been used to help with COPD. To make ginger tea, steep 1-2 teaspoons of sliced fresh

ginger or 1 teaspoon of dried ginger powder in 8 ounces of hot water for 5-10 minutes.

DANDRUFF

1. Sage tea: Sage is an herb that has been traditionally used to help with dandruff and other scalp conditions. To make sage tea, steep 1-2 teaspoons of dried sage leaves in 8 ounces of hot water for 5-10 minutes. (Sage is also a great herb for hot flashes and night sweats).

2. Rosemary tea: Rosemary is an herb that has been traditionally used to help with dandruff and other scalp conditions. To make rosemary tea, steep 1-2 teaspoons of dried rosemary leaves in 8 ounces of hot water for 5-10 minutes.

3. Nettle tea: Nettle is used to help with allergies and to support overall health. It has also been used to help with dandruff. To make nettle tea, steep 1-2 teaspoons of dried nettle leaves in 8 ounces of hot water for 5-10 minutes.

4. Peppermint tea: Peppermint is a refreshing herb that helps with digestion and headaches. It has also been used to help with dandruff. To make peppermint tea, steep 1-2 teaspoons of dried peppermint leaves in 8 ounces of hot water for 5-10 minutes.

5. Chamomile tea: Chamomile is a calming herb which means it is great for sleep and relaxation - it is also very easy to grow - but it is also used to help with dandruff. To make chamomile tea, steep 1-2 teaspoons of dried chamomile flowers in 8 ounces of hot water for 5-10 minutes.

DEPRESSION

1. St. John's wort tea: St. John's wort is often used to ease depression and anxiety. To make St. John's wort tea, steep 1-2 teaspoons of dried St. John's wort in 8 ounces of hot water for 5-10 minutes. St. John's wort flower tea can be made by bringing a pot of water to a boil (about eight ounces) and adding a teaspoon of the flowers (dried or fresh). Steep for 3-8 minutes, then filter out the flowers. You can add honey, but milk or sugar might alter the medicinal effects. Don't take it internally without checking with a health professional.

2. Lemon balm tea: Lemon balm is an herb that has been traditionally used to help with anxiety and to improve sleep. It has also been used to help with depression. To make lemon balm tea, steep 1-2 teaspoons of dried lemon balm leaves in 8 ounces of hot water for 5-10 minutes.

3. Chamomile tea: Chamomile is a calming herb that has been traditionally used to help with sleep and relaxation. It has also been used to help with depression. To make chamomile tea, steep 1-2 teaspoons of dried chamomile flowers in 8 ounces of hot water for 5-10 minutes.

4. Lavender tea: Lavender is an herb that has been traditionally used to help with relaxation and to improve sleep. It has also been used to help with depression. To make lavender tea, steep 1-2 teaspoons of dried lavender flowers in 8 ounces of hot water for 5-10 minutes.

5. Valerian root tea: Valerian root is an herb that has been traditionally used to help with anxiety and to improve

sleep. It has also been used to help with depression. To make valerian root tea, steep 1-2 teaspoons of dried valerian root in 8 ounces of hot water for 5-10 minutes.

DIABETES

Here are a few herbal tea recipes that may help with diabetes:

1. Bitter melon tea: To make bitter melon tea, steep 1-2 teaspoons of dried bitter melon in 8 ounces of hot water for 5-10 minutes.
2. Fenugreek tea: Steep 1-2 teaspoons of dried fenugreek seeds in 8 ounces of hot water for 5-10 minutes.
3. Holy basil tea: Holy basil is an herb that has been traditionally used to help with diabetes. To make holy basil tea, steep 1-2 teaspoons of dried holy basil leaves in 8 ounces of hot water for 5-10 minutes.
4. Gymnema tea: Gymnema is another herb that has been traditionally used to help with diabetes. To make gymnema tea, steep 1-2 teaspoons of dried gymnema leaves in 8 ounces of hot water for 5-10 minutes.
5. Cinnamon tea: Cinnamon is an herb that can be added to other teas or can made as by itself to help diabetes. To make cinnamon tea, steep 1-2 teaspoons of cinnamon bark or cinnamon powder in 8 ounces of hot water for 5-10 minutes. If you are using fresh cinnamon then either add 2 whole ticks to your brew or break it into smaller piece (you can slice it too) before pouring your boiling water over it (not forgetting to strain at the end!). In this example you can add honey or lemon to taste. Cinnamon can have a strong flavor, so you may want to start with a small amount and adjust to taste.

DIARRHEA

Here are a few herbal tea recipes that may help to reduce symptoms of diarrhea:

1. Chamomile tea: Chamomile, with its calming effect on the digestive system, can help to reduce symptoms of diarrhea. To make chamomile tea, steep one teaspoon of dried chamomile flowers in one cup of boiling water for 5-10 minutes. Strain and drink one cup of the tea per day.

2. Peppermint tea: Peppermint is a herb that has been shown to improve digestion and reduce symptoms of diarrhea. To make peppermint tea, steep one teaspoon of dried peppermint leaves in one cup of boiling water for 5-10 minutes. Strain and drink one cup of the tea per day.

3. Slippery elm tea: Slippery elm is a herb that is believed to coat the lining of the digestive tract and may help to reduce symptoms of diarrhea. To make slippery elm tea, steep one teaspoon of slippery elm bark in one cup of boiling water for 5-10 minutes. Strain and drink one cup of the tea per day.

4. Marshmallow root tea: Marshmallow root is another herb that is believed to coat the lining of the digestive tract and can help reduce symptoms of diarrhea. To make marshmallow root tea, steep one teaspoon of dried marshmallow root in one cup of boiling water for 5-10 minutes. Strain and drink one cup of the tea per day.

DRY COUGH

- Marshmallow root tea: Marshmallow root is a herb that is believed to have mucilage properties, which may help to soothe a dry cough. To make marshmallow root tea, steep one teaspoon of dried marshmallow root in one cup of boiling water for 5-10 minutes. Strain and drink one cup of the tea several times per day.
- Licorice root tea: Licorice root is a herb that is believed to have expectorant properties, which may help to relieve a dry cough. To make licorice root tea, steep one teaspoon of dried licorice root in one cup of boiling water for 5-10 minutes. Strain and drink one cup of the tea several times per day.
- Thyme tea: Thyme is another herb that has natural expectorant properties and can relieve a dry cough. To make thyme tea, steep one teaspoon of dried thyme leaves in one cup of boiling water for 5-10 minutes. Strain and drink one cup of the tea several times per day.
- Mullein tea: Mullein is also herb that has natural expectorant properties that may help relieve a dry cough. To make mullein tea, steep one teaspoon of dried mullein leaves in one cup of boiling water for 5-10 minutes. Strain and drink one cup of the tea several times per day.

DRY SKIN

Here are a few herbal tea recipes that may help with dry skin:

1. Calendula tea: Calendula is an herb that has been traditionally used to help with skin irritation and inflammation. To make calendula tea, steep 1-2 teaspoons of dried calendula flowers in 8 ounces of hot water for 5-10 minutes.

2. Chamomile tea: Chamomile is a calming herb that helps with sleep and relaxation. It has also been used to help with dry skin. To make chamomile tea, steep 1-2 teaspoons of dried chamomile flowers in 8 ounces of hot water for 5-10 minutes.

3. Lavender tea: Lavender is an herb that is used to help with relaxation and to improve sleep. It has also been used to help with dry skin. To make lavender tea, steep 1-2 teaspoons of dried lavender flowers in 8 ounces of hot water for 5-10 minutes.

4. Nettle tea: Nettle is an herb that is known to help with allergies and to support overall health. It has also been used to help with dry skin. To make nettle tea, steep 1-2 teaspoons of dried nettle leaves in 8 ounces of hot water for 5-10 minutes.

5. Almond milk tea: Almond milk is a natural moisturizer that has been traditionally used to help with dry skin. To make almond milk tea, combine 1 cup of unsweetened almond milk, 1 cup of water, and 1-2 teaspoons of your favorite tea leaves in a saucepan. Bring to a boil, then reduce the heat and let it simmer for 5-10 minutes. Strain the tea and enjoy.

ECZEMA

1. Chamomile tea: Chamomile has anti-inflammatory properties and may help to soothe the skin. To make chamomile tea, steep 1-2 teaspoons of dried chamomile flowers in 8 ounces of hot water for 5-10 minutes.
2. Calendula tea: Calendula also has anti-inflammatory properties that can help to soothe the skin. To make calendula tea, steep 1-2 teaspoons of dried calendula flowers in 8 ounces of hot water for 5-10 minutes.
3. Licorice tea: Licorice is an herb that has been traditionally used to help with eczema. It too has anti-inflammatory properties and may help to soothe the skin. To make licorice tea, steep 1-2 teaspoons of dried licorice root in 8 ounces of hot water for 5-10 minutes.
4. Aloe vera tea: Aloe vera, with its moisturizing properties, is an herb that has been used for thousands of years to sooth eczema and calm the skin. To make aloe vera tea, steep 1-2 teaspoons of dried aloe vera leaves in 8 ounces of hot water for 5-10 minutes.
5. Oat straw tea: Oat straw is an herb that also has soothing properties that may help to moisturize the skin. To make oat straw tea, steep 1-2 teaspoons of dried oat straw in 8 ounces of hot water for 5-10 minutes.

FLU

1. Echinacea tea: Echinacea is a herb that is believed to have immune-boosting properties and may help to reduce symptoms of the flu. To make echinacea tea, steep one teaspoon of dried echinacea in one cup of boiling water

for 5-10 minutes. Strain and drink one cup of the tea several times per day.

2. Elderberry tea: Elderberry is another herb that is believed to have immune-boosting properties and may help to reduce symptoms of the flu. To make elderberry tea, steep one teaspoon of dried elderberries in one cup of boiling water for 5-10 minutes. Strain and drink one cup of the tea several times per day.

3. Ginger tea: Ginger is a herb that has natural anti-inflammatory and immune-boosting properties. To make ginger tea, steep one teaspoon of freshly grated ginger in one cup of boiling water for 5-10 minutes. Strain and drink one cup of the tea several times per day.

4. Garlic tea: Garlic - a wonderful herb - has natural immune-boosting properties. To make garlic tea, steep one clove of minced garlic in one cup of boiling water for 5-10 minutes. Strain and drink one cup of the tea several times per day.

GREASY HAIR

1. Rosemary tea: Rosemary is an herb that has been traditionally used to help with dandruff and other scalp conditions. It has also been used to help with greasy hair. To make rosemary tea, steep 1-2 teaspoons of dried rosemary leaves in 8 ounces of hot water for 10-15 minutes.

2. Sage tea: Sage is an herb that has been traditionally used to help with dandruff and other scalp conditions. It has also been used to help with greasy hair. To make sage

tea, steep 1-2 teaspoons of dried sage leaves in 8 ounces of hot water for 5-15 minutes.

3. Peppermint tea: Peppermint is a refreshing herb that has been traditionally used to help with digestion and headaches. It has also been used to help with greasy hair. To make peppermint tea, steep 1-2 teaspoons of dried peppermint leaves in 8 ounces of hot water for 5-10 minutes.

4. Lemon balm tea: Lemon balm is an herb that has been traditionally used to help with anxiety and to improve sleep. It has also been used to help with greasy hair. To make lemon balm tea, steep 1-2 teaspoons of dried lemon balm leaves in 8 ounces of hot water for 5-10 minutes.

5. Nettle tea: Nettle is an herb that has been traditionally used to help with allergies and to support overall health. It has also been used to help with greasy hair. To make nettle tea, steep 1-2 teaspoons of dried nettle leaves in 8 ounces of hot water for 5-10 minutes.

GRIEF

1. Chamomile tea: Chamomile is a herb that has a natural calming effect and may help to reduce feelings of grief. To make chamomile tea, steep one teaspoon of dried chamomile flowers in one cup of boiling water for 5-10 minutes. Strain and drink one cup of the tea several times per day.

2. Lavender tea: Lavender is also a herb that has a natural calming effect and may help to reduce feelings of grief. To make lavender tea, steep one teaspoon of dried

lavender flowers in one cup of boiling water for 5-10 minutes. Strain and drink one cup of the tea several times per day.

3. Lemon balm tea: Lemon balm is another herb that has a natural calming effect and may help to reduce feelings of grief. To make lemon balm tea, steep one teaspoon of dried lemon balm leaves in one cup of boiling water for 5-10 minutes. Strain and drink one cup of the tea several times per day.

4. Valerian root tea: Valerian root has a natural calming effect and may help to reduce feelings of grief. To make valerian root tea, steep one teaspoon of dried valerian root in one cup of boiling water for 5-15 minutes. Strain and drink one cup of the tea several times per day.

GUT HEALTH

1. Chamomile tea: Chamomile has been shown to have a calming effect on the digestive system and may help to reduce symptoms of indigestion and bloating. To make chamomile tea, steep one teaspoon of dried chamomile flowers in one cup of boiling water for 5-10 minutes. Strain and drink one cup of the tea per day.

2. Peppermint tea: Peppermint is a herb that improves digestion and reduces symptoms of indigestion and bloating. To make peppermint tea, steep one teaspoon of dried peppermint leaves in one cup of boiling water for 5-10 minutes. Strain and drink one cup of the tea per day.

3. Ginger tea: Ginger improves digestion and reduce symptoms of nausea. To make ginger tea, steep one

teaspoon of freshly grated ginger in one cup of boiling water for 5-10 minutes. Strain and drink one cup of the tea per day.

4. Fennel tea: Fennel also improves digestion and reduce symptoms of bloating. To make fennel tea, steep one teaspoon of dried fennel seeds in one cup of boiling water for 5-10 minutes. Strain and drink one cup of the tea per day.

HAIR LOSS

There are several herbal teas that may be helpful for hair loss. Here are a few recipes that you can try:

1. Nettle tea: Nettle is a herb that is rich in vitamins and minerals, including silica, which may help to strengthen hair. To make nettle tea, steep one tablespoon of dried nettle leaves in one cup of boiling water for 10-15 minutes. Strain and drink one cup of the tea per day.

2. Sage tea: Sage is a herb that is believed to have hair-strengthening properties. To make sage tea, steep one tablespoon of dried sage leaves in one cup of boiling water for 10-15 minutes. Strain and drink one cup of the tea per day.

3. Rosemary tea: Rosemary is a herb that is thought to improve circulation to the scalp, which may help to stimulate hair growth. To make rosemary tea, steep one tablespoon of dried rosemary leaves in one cup of boiling water for 10-15 minutes. Strain and drink one cup of the tea per day.

4. Green tea: Green tea is rich in antioxidants and is believed to have hair-healthy benefits. To make green

tea, steep one teaspoon of green tea leaves in one cup of boiling water for 2-5 minutes. Strain and drink one cup of the tea per day.

HEADACHE & MIGRAINE

1. Peppermint tea: Peppermint is a refreshing herb that has been traditionally used to help with digestion and headaches. To make peppermint tea, steep 1-2 teaspoons of dried peppermint leaves in 8 ounces of hot water for 5-10 minutes.
2. Ginger tea: Ginger is a warming herb that has been traditionally used to help with nausea and inflammation. It has also been used to help with headaches. To make ginger tea, steep 1-2 teaspoons of sliced fresh ginger or 1 teaspoon of dried ginger powder in 8 ounces of hot water for 2-5 minutes.
3. Chamomile tea: Chamomile is a calming herb that has been traditionally used to help with sleep and relaxation. It has also been used to help with headaches. To make chamomile tea, steep 1-2 teaspoons of dried chamomile flowers in 8 ounces of hot water for 5-10 minutes.
4. Willow bark tea: Willow bark is an herb that has been traditionally used to help with pain and inflammation. It has also been used to help with headaches. To make willow bark tea, steep 1-2 teaspoons of dried willow bark in 8 ounces of hot water for 5-10 minutes.
5. Rosemary tea: Rosemary is an herb that has been traditionally used to help with digestion and to improve memory. It has also been used to help with headaches. To make rosemary tea, steep 1-2 teaspoons of dried

rosemary leaves in 8 ounces of hot water for 5-15 minutes.

6. Feverfew tea: Feverfew is an herb that has been traditionally used to help with migraines and other types of headaches. To make feverfew tea, steep 1-2 teaspoons of dried feverfew leaves in 8 ounces of hot water for 5-10 minutes.

HIGH BLOOD PRESSURE

1. Hibiscus tea: Hibiscus is a herb that has natural diuretic properties and may help to reduce high blood pressure. To make hibiscus tea, steep one teaspoon of dried hibiscus flowers in one cup of boiling water for 5-10 minutes. Strain and drink one cup of the tea several times per day.

2. Garlic tea: Garlic is a herb that has natural anti-inflammatory and blood pressure-lowering properties and may help to reduce high blood pressure. To make garlic tea, steep one clove of minced garlic in one cup of boiling water for 5-10 minutes. Strain and drink one cup of the tea several times per day.

3. Hawthorn tea: Hawthorn is a herb that is believed to have blood pressure-lowering properties and may help to reduce high blood pressure. To make hawthorn tea, steep one teaspoon of dried hawthorn berries in one cup of boiling water for 5-10 minutes. Strain and drink one cup of the tea several times per day.

4. Basil tea: Basil is a herb that has natural anti-inflammatory properties and may help to reduce high blood pressure. To make basil tea, steep one teaspoon of

dried basil leaves in one cup of boiling water for 5-10 minutes. Strain and drink one cup of the tea several times per day.

IMPROVE FOCUS

1. Peppermint tea: Peppermint is a herb that has been shown to improve focus and concentration. To make peppermint tea, steep one teaspoon of dried peppermint leaves in one cup of boiling water for 5-10 minutes. Strain and drink one cup of the tea per day.
2. Rosemary tea: Rosemary is a herb that is believed to improve focus and cognitive function. To make rosemary tea, steep one teaspoon of dried rosemary leaves in one cup of boiling water for 5-15 minutes. Strain and drink one cup of the tea per day.
3. Ginkgo biloba tea: Ginkgo biloba is a herb that is believed to improve blood flow to the brain, which may help to improve focus and concentration. To make ginkgo biloba tea, steep one teaspoon of dried ginkgo biloba leaves in one cup of boiling water for 5-10 minutes. Strain and drink one cup of the tea per day.
4. Green tea: Green tea is rich in antioxidants and is believed to have brain-healthy benefits. To make green tea, steep one teaspoon of green tea leaves in one cup of boiling water for 2-5 minutes. Strain and drink one cup of the tea per day.

IMPROVE MEMORY

1. Rosemary tea: Rosemary is a herb that has been shown to improve memory and cognitive function. To make rosemary tea, steep one teaspoon of dried rosemary leaves in one cup of boiling water for 5-15 minutes. Strain and drink one cup of the tea per day.
2. Ginkgo biloba tea: Ginkgo biloba is a herb that is believed to improve blood flow to the brain, which may help to improve memory and cognitive function. To make ginkgo biloba tea, steep one teaspoon of dried ginkgo biloba leaves in one cup of boiling water for 5-10 minutes. Strain and drink one cup of the tea per day.
3. Brahmi tea: Brahmi is an Ayurvedic herb that is believed to improve memory and cognitive function. To make brahmi tea, steep one teaspoon of dried brahmi leaves in one cup of boiling water for 5-10 minutes. Strain and drink one cup of the tea per day.
4. Green tea: Green tea is rich in antioxidants and is believed to have brain-healthy benefits. To make green tea, steep one teaspoon of green tea leaves in one cup of boiling water for 2-5 minutes. Strain and drink one cup of the tea per day.

IRRITABLE BOWEL SYNDROME (IBS)

Here are a some herbal tea recipes to try that may help with IBS:

1. Peppermint tea: Peppermint is a refreshing herb that has been traditionally used to help with digestion and headaches. It has also been used to help with IBS. To

make peppermint tea, steep 1-2 teaspoons of dried peppermint leaves in 8 ounces of hot water for 5-10 minutes.

2. Chamomile tea: Chamomile is a calming herb that has been traditionally used to help with sleep and relaxation. It has also been used to help with IBS. To make chamomile tea, steep 1-2 teaspoons of dried chamomile flowers in 8 ounces of hot water for 5-10 minutes.

3. Fennel tea: Fennel is an herb that has been traditionally used to help with digestion and bloating. It has also been used to help with IBS. To make fennel tea, steep 1-2 teaspoons of dried fennel seeds in 8 ounces of hot water for 5-10 minutes.

4. Ginger tea: Ginger is a warming herb that has been traditionally used to help with nausea and inflammation. It has also been used to help with IBS. To make ginger tea, steep 1-2 teaspoons of sliced fresh ginger or 1 teaspoon of dried ginger powder in 8 ounces of hot water for 5-10 minutes.

5. Licorice tea: Licorice is an herb that has been traditionally used to help with digestive issues and to soothe the throat. It has also been used to help with IBS. To make licorice tea, steep 1-2 teaspoons of dried licorice root in 8 ounces of hot water for 5-15 minutes.

If you have IBS then try to avoid senna, rhubarb root and buckthorn bark tea which, although generally good for the digestive system, are all natural laxatives that can cause cramping, bloating, and diarrhea, and can worsen IBS symptoms.

LOW BLOOD PRESSURE

Here are a few herbal tea recipes that may help to increase low blood pressure:

1. Licorice root tea: Licorice root is a herb that is believed to have blood pressure-increasing properties and may help to increase low blood pressure. To make licorice root tea, steep one teaspoon of dried licorice root in one cup of boiling water for 5-15 minutes. Strain and drink one cup of the tea several times per day.

2. Ginger tea: Ginger is a herb that has natural blood pressure-increasing properties and may help to increase low blood pressure. To make ginger tea, steep one teaspoon of freshly grated ginger in one cup of boiling water for 5-10 minutes. Strain and drink one cup of the tea several times per day.

3. Cinnamon tea: Cinnamon is a herb that is believed to have blood pressure-increasing properties and may help to increase low blood pressure. To make cinnamon tea, steep one teaspoon of cinnamon bark in one cup of boiling water for 5-10 minutes. Strain and drink one cup of the tea several times per day.

4. Cardamom tea: Cardamom is a herb that is believed to have blood pressure-increasing properties and may help to increase low blood pressure. To make cardamom tea, steep one teaspoon of cardamom seeds in one cup of boiling water for 5-10 minutes. Strain and drink one cup of the tea several times per day.

MENOPAUSE

Here are a few herbal tea recipes that may help with menopause:

1. Red clover tea: Red clover is an herb that has been traditionally used to help with menopause symptoms such as hot flashes and night sweats. To make red clover tea, steep 1-2 teaspoons of dried red clover flowers in 8 ounces of hot water for 5-10 minutes.
2. Black cohosh tea: Black cohosh is an herb that has been traditionally used to help with menopause symptoms such as hot flashes and mood changes. To make black cohosh tea, steep 1-2 teaspoons of dried black cohosh root in 8 ounces of hot water for 5-10 minutes.
3. Sage tea: Sage is an herb that has been traditionally used to help with menopause symptoms such as hot flashes and night sweats. To make sage tea, steep 1-2 teaspoons of dried sage leaves in 8 ounces of hot water for 5-15 minutes.
4. Wild yam tea: Wild yam is an herb that has been traditionally used to help with menopause symptoms such as hot flashes and mood changes. To make wild yam tea, steep 1-2 teaspoons of dried wild yam root in 8 ounces of hot water for 5-10 minutes.
5. Chasteberry tea: Chasteberry is an herb that has been traditionally used to help with menopause symptoms such as hot flashes and mood changes. To make chasteberry tea, steep 1-2 teaspoons of dried chasteberry in 8 ounces of hot water for 5-10 minutes.

MENSTRUAL PAIN

1. Chamomile tea: Chamomile is a herb that has natural pain-relieving and anti-inflammatory properties and may help to reduce symptoms of menstrual pain. To make chamomile tea, steep one teaspoon of dried chamomile flowers in one cup of boiling water for 5-10 minutes. Strain and drink one cup of the tea several times per day.

2. Ginger tea: Ginger is a herb that has natural pain-relieving and anti-inflammatory properties and may help to reduce symptoms of menstrual pain. To make ginger tea, steep one teaspoon of freshly grated ginger in one cup of boiling water for 5-10 minutes. Strain and drink one cup of the tea several times per day.

3. Peppermint tea: Peppermint is a herb that has natural pain-relieving and anti-inflammatory properties and may help to reduce symptoms of menstrual pain. To make peppermint tea, steep one teaspoon of dried peppermint leaves in one cup of boiling water for 5-10 minutes. Strain and drink one cup of the tea several times per day.

4. Fennel tea: Fennel is a herb that has natural pain-relieving and anti-inflammatory properties and may help to reduce symptoms of menstrual pain. To make fennel tea, steep one teaspoon of dried fennel seeds in one cup of boiling water for 5-10 minutes. Strain and drink one cup of the tea several times per day.

MOTIVATION AND ENERGY

1. Green tea: Green tea is a type of tea that contains caffeine and may help to increase motivation and energy. To make green tea, steep one teaspoon of green tea leaves in one cup of boiling water for 2-5 minutes. Strain and drink one cup of the tea in the morning or as needed for a boost of energy.

2. Yerba mate tea: Yerba mate is a type of tea that contains caffeine and may help to increase motivation and energy. To make yerba mate tea, steep one teaspoon of yerba mate leaves in one cup of boiling water for 5-10 minutes. Strain and drink one cup of the tea in the morning or as needed for a boost of energy.

3. Guarana tea: Guarana is a herb that contains caffeine and may help to increase motivation and energy. To make guarana tea, steep one teaspoon of guarana powder in one cup of boiling water for 5-10 minutes. Strain and drink one cup of the tea in the morning or as needed for a boost of energy.

4. Ginkgo biloba tea: Ginkgo biloba is a herb that is believed to improve mental clarity and may help to increase motivation and energy. To make ginkgo biloba tea, steep one teaspoon of ginkgo biloba leaves in one cup of boiling water for 5-10 minutes. Strain and drink one cup of the tea in the morning or as needed for a boost of energy.

PSORIASIS

1. Burdock tea: Burdock is an herb that has been traditionally used to help with psoriasis. It has anti-inflammatory properties and may help to reduce skin irritation. To make burdock tea, steep 1-2 teaspoons of dried burdock root in 8 ounces of hot water for 5-10 minutes.

2. Calendula tea: Calendula is an herb that has been traditionally used to help with psoriasis. It has anti-inflammatory properties and may help to reduce skin irritation. To make calendula tea, steep 1-2 teaspoons of dried calendula flowers in 8 ounces of hot water for 5-10 minutes.

3. Licorice tea: Licorice is an herb that has been traditionally used to help with psoriasis. It has anti-inflammatory properties and may help to reduce skin irritation. To make licorice tea, steep 1-2 teaspoons of dried licorice root in 8 ounces of hot water for 5-10 minutes.

4. Aloe vera tea: Aloe vera is an herb that has been traditionally used to help with psoriasis. It has moisturizing properties and may help to soothe the skin. To make aloe vera tea, steep 1-2 teaspoons of dried aloe vera leaves in 8 ounces of hot water for 5-10 minutes.

5. Oat straw tea: Oat straw is an herb that has been traditionally used to help with psoriasis. It has soothing properties and may help to moisturize the skin. To make oat straw tea, steep 1-2 teaspoons of dried oat straw in 8 ounces of hot water for 5-10 minutes.

SLEEP

1. Chamomile tea: Chamomile is a herb that has a natural calming effect and may help to improve sleep. To make chamomile tea, steep one teaspoon of dried chamomile flowers in one cup of boiling water for 5-10 minutes. Strain and drink one cup of the tea an hour before bedtime. Like many herbal teas you can add honey or lemon (optional)

2. Lavender tea: Lavender is a herb that has a natural calming effect and may help to improve sleep. To make lavender tea, steep one teaspoon of dried lavender flowers in one cup of boiling water for 5-10 minutes. Strain and drink one cup of the tea an hour before bedtime.

3. Valerian root tea: Valerian root is a herb that has a natural calming effect and may help to improve sleep. To make valerian root tea, steep one teaspoon of dried valerian root in one cup of boiling water for 5-10 minutes. Strain and drink one cup of the tea an hour before bedtime.

4. Lemon balm tea: Lemon balm is a herb that has a natural calming effect and may help to improve sleep. To make lemon balm tea, steep one teaspoon of dried lemon balm leaves in one cup of boiling water for 5-10 minutes. Strain and drink one cup of the tea an hour before bedtime.

SORE THROAT

1. Chamomile tea: Chamomile is a herb that has a natural pain-relieving and anti-inflammatory effect and may help to reduce symptoms of a sore throat. To make chamomile tea, steep one teaspoon of dried chamomile flowers in one cup of boiling water for 5-10 minutes. Strain and drink one cup of the tea several times per day.
2. Peppermint tea: Peppermint is a herb that has a natural pain-relieving and anti-inflammatory effect and may help to reduce symptoms of a sore throat. To make peppermint tea, steep one teaspoon of dried peppermint leaves in one cup of boiling water for 5-10 minutes. Strain and drink one cup of the tea several times per day.
3. Marshmallow root tea: Marshmallow root is a herb that is believed to coat the throat and may help to reduce symptoms of a sore throat. To make marshmallow root tea, steep one teaspoon of dried marshmallow root in one cup of boiling water for 5-10 minutes. Strain and drink one cup of the tea several times per day.
4. Licorice root tea: Licorice root is a herb that is believed to coat the throat and may help to reduce symptoms of a sore throat. To make licorice root tea, steep one teaspoon of dried licorice root in one cup of boiling water for 5-15 minutes. Strain and drink one cup of the tea several times per day.

STOMACH HEALTH

1. Chamomile tea: Chamomile is a calming herb that has been traditionally used to help with sleep and relaxation.

It has also been used to help with digestive issues. To make chamomile tea, steep 1-2 teaspoons of dried chamomile flowers in 8 ounces of hot water for 5-10 minutes.

2. Ginger tea: Ginger is a warming herb that has been traditionally used to help with nausea and inflammation. To make ginger tea, steep 1-2 teaspoons of sliced fresh ginger or 1 teaspoon of dried ginger powder in 8 ounces of hot water for 5-10 minutes.

3. Peppermint tea: Peppermint is a refreshing herb that has been traditionally used to help with digestion and headaches. To make peppermint tea, steep 1-2 teaspoons of dried peppermint leaves in 8 ounces of hot water for 5-10 minutes.

4. Fennel tea: Fennel is an herb that has been traditionally used to help with digestion and bloating. To make fennel tea, steep 1-2 teaspoons of dried fennel seeds in 8 ounces of hot water for 5-10 minutes.

5. Licorice tea: Licorice is an herb that has been traditionally used to help with digestive issues and to soothe the throat. To make licorice tea, steep 1-2 teaspoons of dried licorice root in 8 ounces of hot water for 5-15 minutes.

TOOTHACHE

1. Chamomile tea: Chamomile is a herb that has a natural pain-relieving effect and may help to reduce toothache pain. To make chamomile tea, steep one teaspoon of dried chamomile flowers in one cup of boiling water for 5-10 minutes. Strain and use the cooled tea as a mouth rinse.

2. Clove tea: Clove is a herb that has a natural pain-relieving and antibacterial effect and may help to reduce toothache pain. To make clove tea, steep one teaspoon of dried clove buds in one cup of boiling water for 5-10 minutes. Strain and use the cooled tea as a mouth rinse.

3. Peppermint tea: Peppermint is a herb that has a natural pain-relieving and antibacterial effect and may help to reduce toothache pain. To make peppermint tea, steep one teaspoon of dried peppermint leaves in one cup of boiling water for 5-10 minutes. Strain and use the cooled tea as a mouth rinse.

4. Ginger tea: Ginger is a herb that has a natural pain-relieving effect and may help to reduce toothache pain. To make ginger tea, steep one teaspoon of freshly grated ginger in one cup of boiling water for 5-10 minutes. Strain and use the cooled tea as a mouth rinse.

Instructions for clove tea

- Place the clove buds in a tea infuser or wrap them in a piece of cheesecloth.
- Place the tea infuser or cheesecloth with the clove buds in a cup.
- Pour the boiling water over the clove buds.
- Allow the tea to steep for 5-10 minutes.
- Remove the tea infuser or cheesecloth with the clove buds.
- Drink the tea while it is still warm.

Clove tea is a herbal tea made from the dried buds of the clove plant. It has a warm, spicy flavor and has natural pain-relieving and antibacterial properties. It is also believed to have digestive and immune-boosting benefits.

UTI (URINARY TRACT INFECTION)

1. Cranberry tea: Cranberry is an herb that has been traditionally used to help with UTI. It has antibacterial properties and may help to prevent the growth of bacteria in the urinary tract. To make cranberry tea, steep 1-2 teaspoons of dried cranberry in 8 ounces of hot water for 5-10 minutes.

2. Dandelion tea: Dandelion is an herb that has been traditionally used to help with UTI. It has diuretic properties and may help to flush toxins from the body. To make dandelion tea, steep 1-2 teaspoons of dried dandelion leaves in 8 ounces of hot water for 5-10 minutes.

3. Uva ursi tea: Uva ursi is an herb that has been traditionally used to help with UTI. It has antimicrobial properties and may help to reduce the growth of bacteria in the urinary tract. To make uva ursi tea, steep 1-2 teaspoons of dried uva ursi leaves in 8 ounces of hot water for 5-10 minutes.

4. Bearberry tea: Bearberry is an herb that has been traditionally used to help with UTI. It has antimicrobial properties and may help to reduce the growth of bacteria in the urinary tract. To make bearberry tea, steep 1-2 teaspoons of dried bearberry leaves in 8 ounces of hot water for 5-10 minutes.

5. Corn silk tea: Corn silk is an herb that has been traditionally used to help with UTI. It has diuretic

properties and may help to flush toxins from the body. To make corn silk tea, steep 1-2 teaspoons of dried corn silk in 8 ounces of hot water for 5-10 minutes.

YEAST INFECTION

1. Cranberry tea: Cranberry is an herb that has been traditionally used to help with yeast infections. It has antibacterial properties and may help to prevent the growth of bacteria in the urinary tract. To make cranberry tea, steep 1-2 teaspoons of dried cranberry in 8 ounces of hot water for 5-10 minutes.

2. Garlic tea: Garlic is an herb that has been traditionally used to help with yeast infections. It has antimicrobial properties and may help to reduce the growth of yeast in the body. To make garlic tea, steep 1-2 cloves of sliced fresh garlic in 8 ounces of hot water for 5-10 minutes.

3. Oregano tea: Oregano is an herb that has been traditionally used to help with yeast infections. It has antimicrobial properties and may help to reduce the growth of yeast in the body. To make oregano tea, steep 1-2 teaspoons of dried oregano leaves in 8 ounces of hot water for 5-10 minutes.

4. Thyme tea: Thyme is an herb that has been traditionally used to help with yeast infections. It has antimicrobial properties and may help to reduce the growth of yeast in the body. To make thyme tea, steep 1-2 teaspoons of dried thyme leaves in 8 ounces of hot water for 5-10 minutes.

5. Calendula tea: Calendula is an herb that has been traditionally used to help with yeast infections. It has

anti-inflammatory properties and may help to reduce skin irritation. To make calendula tea, steep 1-2 teaspoons of dried calendula flowers in 8 ounces of hot water for 5-10 minutes.

CHAPTER 6

12 herbs and what they are good for

As you can see from the previous chapters, making herbal tea does not need to be complicated and, in fact, is very straight-forward.

The most important part of the process is knowing which herb to use and why you need that herb.

In this chapter I have provided an example of the details of 12 of the herbs covered in this that book that you may already have in your kitchen. It should give you a better idea of the importance of these herbs and will help indicate what you can find out Along with each herbs are some more tea recipes mixes.

BASIL

There has been a great deal of research into the effects of basil. The essential oil and eugenol that basil contains have been proven to help fight inflammation in the body, lowering the risk of inflammatory issues such as arthritis, heart disease, and bowel issues.

In 2001 researchers were also able to link the properties of sweet basil (as an extract) to aging when their findings suggested that it might help protect the skin from some of the effects.

The most considerable body of evidence revolves around the antioxidant properties of basil. It contains flavonoids, such as orientin and vicenin, and these can help protect against cell damage and protect against health conditions, including cancer, heart disease, arthritis, and diabetes.

Basil is also a calming adaptogen which means that it is great for reducing stress.

The most effective compounds can disappear during the drying process, so use fresh basil whenever possible for the most benefit.

To make tea, add 2 tablespoons of finely chopped basil to a saucepan and add a little ginger. Add a cup of boiling water and then steep for a round 5 minutes. Strain and pour. You add lemon and honey to taste.

What it's good for:

- Anti-oxidant
- Can protect skin against aging
- Can reduce cholesterol and protect against heart disease
- Anti-bacterial
- Anti-inflammatory

- Can improve mental health and focus
- Improves digestion
- Good for colds
- Improves liver function
- Reduces mucus

CALENDULA

Calendula has a mildly sweet and bitter taste and contains several potent antioxidants, including triterpenes, flavonoids, polyphenols, and carotenoids, and the flower that is the medicinal part of the plant.

According to *Healthline* a study of rats fed monosodium glutamate (MSG), calendula extract significantly reduced oxidative stress and reverted the depletion of antioxidant levels by up to 122%.

Other studies have suggested that the extract has antiviral and anti-inflammatory properties.

It has traditionally been used for abdominal cramps and constipation, and tests have shown some evidence for this use due to its spasmogenic effects.

Although the Food and Drug Administration (FDA) considers calendula safe for general use, it can cause allergic reactions and like many herbs and remedies, should be avoided during pregnancy (and given its possible menstruation effects).

The tea can soothe sore throats or any internal mucous membranes, including the intestinal tract and gut, and help digestion.

To make tea, boil your water, then add it to your infuser or teapot, which contains two teaspoons of dried calendula flowers. Leave for ten minutes, strain, and drink. You can add any flavoring, including cinnamon or honey (or both!)

The tea can either be drunk or used to help sunburns, rashes, or sores.

What it's good for:

- Anticancer
- Anti-diabetic
- Antofungal (candida)
- Anti-inflammatory
- Antioxidant
- Antimicrobial
- Antiviral
- Prevents blood from clotting
- Neuro protective
- Sore throats/mouth/mucous membranes
- Urinary tract infections
- Relieve treatment-related side effects of cancer
- May protect against sunburn

CHAMOMILE

Chamomile contains more than 120 chemical parts, including active apigenin and luteolin, and it contains flavonoids and small amounts of coumarin, which may have some mild blood-thinning effects.

As well as helping your central nervous system, chamomile is also great for your Enteric Nervous System, which controls your gut. It calms your gut and is particularly good if you tend to hold stress in your digestive system.

Interestingly, the evidence of its efficacy as a sleep inducer is not conclusive, probably due to the lack of robust human tests, but there is evidence that it can help to reduce anxiety and stress and may be an anit-depressant and anti-inflammatory.

Tests in animals also show that it may help diarrhea because it helps to balance the muscle spasms that cause gastrointestinal inflammation, possibly helping bowel disease, but more tests are required.

It is a gentle herb that is safe for most children and adults and can generally used liberally and frequently. It can even be used on dogs if they have an eye infection.

It could interact with other sedatives, blood thinners, antiplatelet drugs, aspirin, NSAID painkillers (ibuprofen and naproxen), and may also interact with supplements like Garlic, St. John's Wort, and Valerian.

Talk to your physician if you are taking other drugs.

Most commonly used to make tea, it can be added to apple dishes such as apple pies.

To make tea - add boiling water to your infuser or teapot that contains one teaspoon of dried or two teaspoons of fresh flowers and brew for five to ten minutes.

It pairs well with ginger for digestive problems, but it takes longer to activate the bitter action meaning that you need to infuse the tea for up to 10-20 minutes.

It is wonderful at relieving stress and should be taken regularly - ideally with rosemary or cinnamon, and you can add one of these to your infusion.

For sleep, add hawthorn berries or ashwagandha (or both).

What it's good for:

- Anti-allergenic
- Anti-inflammatory

- Antimicrobial
- Anti-spasmodic
- Acid Reflux
- Cramping
- Constipation
- Diarrhea
- Digestion (especially stomach, liver and bowel)
- Eye and mouth complaints
- Headaches
- Immune boosting
- Indigestion
- Menstration
- Nausea and vomitting
- Sedative/Insomnia/relaxation/reduce stress and anxiety
- Skin irritations, lesions, bites, stings, wound healing

CILANTRO/CORRIANDER

Cilantro and Coriander (the seeds are often know as Corriander rather than the plant which is known as Cilantro), is packed with antioxidants, which are thought to help reduce inflammation by suppressing inflammation-inducing free radicals.

One animal study found antioxidants in Cilantro extract helped protect the skin from aging, and other studies found that the antioxidants in coriander seed extract could reduce inflammation and inhibit cancer growth in the stomach, prostrate, colon, breast, and lungs.

Cilantro extract may also reduce the formation of blood clots, potentially reducing the risk of heart disease. At the same time, studies have also found that seed extract 'significantly' lowers blood pressure while also encouraging the release of urine which contains salt.

Cilantro leaves were found to be nearly as effective as a diabetes medication at reducing blood sugar levels.

Coriander seeds have been shown to support healthy blood sugar levels and arterial and cardiovascular health and contain antimicrobial, antioxidant, and detoxifying qualities.

For tea, steep a tablespoon of leaves in a cup of hot water and flavor with a pinch of raw honey. Add cilantro seeds to boost the cooling properties.

To use the seeds for tea, steep a teaspoon of whole cilantro seeds in a cup of hot water and flavor it with either raw honey (or orange peel or lime peel).

What it's good for:

- Anti-bacterial
- Anti-inflammatory
- Anti-oxidant
- Anti-fungal
- Antimicrobial
- Anti-viral
- Antiseptic
- Detoxifier (leaves)
- Digestion (indigestion, bloating, gas and cramps)
- Fighting food-borne infections
- Halitosis (bad breath)
- Lower blood pressure (seed extract)
- Natural food preservative
- Promotes skin health
- Reduce blood clots
- Sedative, relaxant and mild laxative
- Urinary tract infections

- Weight loss
- May inhibit the growth of cancer cells

ECHINACEA/CONEFLOWER

Echinacea has a sharp, acrid taste that first hits the mouth and throat, promoting saliva production before dispersing around the body, stimulating the immune system, and triggering lymph flow to the lymphatic glands.

A 2015 analysis of six studies reported evidence to suggest that echinacea may reduce the risk of a reoccurring respiratory infection and the associated complications.

It activates chemicals that decrease inflammation and boost the immune system (it is not an antibiotic - it works through innate immunity rather than antibody-acquired immunity). The immune response focuses, as noted above, on the throat and lymphatic tissues. This makes it good for upper respiratory problems including cold, flu, tonsillitis, pharyngitis, laryngitis, and general mucous and sinus congestion including wound healing, bites and allergies. It is also effective as a mouthwash for gum disease and skin conditions like eczema. It helps soothe toothache, ulcers, and infections of the oral mucous membranes (the mouth).

Because it is good for bacterial-induced inflammation, used internally and externally, it has been shown to help people with recurring boils, acne, and skin abscesses.

Although it is safe for most people, it can have side effects, including stomach pain, nausea, headache, and dizziness. It should not be taken by those who take immunosuppressants or tamoxifen and should be avoided if auto-immune disorders are present (such as multiple sclerosis, lupus, or rheumatoid arthritis).

Echinacea tea can be made from the roots, leaves, flowers, and stems, but the purple flowers and roots are usually used to brew teas.

Bring a pot of water to a boil (about 8-10 ounces of water), turn it down to a simmer, and add one tablespoon of dried echinacea (or two of fresh) and cook for 5-10 minutes. Strain, and then it's ready.

If you are making it in a cup, just pour boiling water into the cup, add the echinacea to a tea infuser, and steep for 5-10 minutes.

You can add honey or lemon to taste. Drink or gargle no more than three times a day.

What it's good for:

- Acne
- Anti-inflammatory
- Antimicrobial
- Boils and ulcers
- Upper respiratory infections
- Gum disease and toothache
- Cold and flu
- Indigestion
- Dizziness and migraines
- UTIs, yeast infections
- Fatigue
- Eczema
- Psoriasis
- Tonsillitis, pharyngitis, laryngitis
- Wound healing

GARLIC

Garlic has over 40 healthy compounds, including flavonoids, arginine, and selenium. The Allicin oil produced when garlic is crushed is a powerful antibiotic, antibacterial and anti-fungal, and it is Allicin that gives garlic its distinctive smell.

There are numerous studies on the health and cardiovascular benefits of garlic. It may help people with heart disease, lower the risk of stroke, lower cholesterol and blood pressure and help prevent blood clots. It also lowers blood sugar levels in those with diabetes.

As an antiviral, garlic is effective against several flu viruses as well as other viruses, including rhinovirus.

Its antibacterial properties are effective against bacteria, including salmonella and E-coli as well as gut bacteria.

Garlic's antioxidant properties mean it is also effective at reducing oxidative stress by fighting the free radicals that cause it which means that may help improve cognition, including managing and preventing dementia and Alzheimer's disease.

As well as all of these benefits, garlic can help detoxify the liver and boost the immune system, which is why it can reduce both the frequency and severity of illnesses like the common cold.

It contains flavonoids, phytochemicals, Vitamin C and B6, manganese, and selenium. It has historically been used to treat dysentery, pneumonia, tuberculosis, asthma, hay fever, diarrhea, snake bites, warts, abscesses, and hepatitis.

For poison ivy, poison oak, and sting nettle make a tea out of garlic and apply when cooled to the affected area (4 cups chopped garlic cloves for each cup of water).

What it's good for:

- Anti-oxidant
- Anti-inflammatory
- Anti-cancer agent
- Antimicrobial

- Bone health
- Detoxifying
- Digestive
- Eye health
- Possibly osteoporosis
- Lowers blood pressure
- Diuretic
- Bloating
- Stimulates metabolism and circulation
- Good for cardiac health.
- Known to help nervousness, anxiety, insomnia, and weight loss
- Encourages sweating (eliminating toxins)

GINGER

There have been many studies on Ginger and its effects.

Studies with cholesterol show that participants experienced drops in total cholesterol and there is also some evidence that ginger can help enhance brain function directly.

Numerous studies in animals show that ginger can help protect against age-related decline in brain function.

There are lots of tea's that you can make with ginger.

Cinnamon clove and ginger tea is good for coughs and clearing the pathways (ginger is an expectorant) and ginger is great for nausea and digestion (and sometimes used for those with sea sickness).

To make a cup of ginger tea, thinly slice a 1 inch piece of ginger (you can leave the peel on), add to a pot of water and bring to boil then reduce to a simmer (five to ten minutes), then strain. You can add a slice of lemon after cooking (or a clove during cooking) and serve with a little honey if you want to sweeten.

. . .

What it's good for:

- Anti-Oxidant
- Anti-Inflammatory
- Anti-diabetic
- Anti-bacterial
- Immuno-nutrition (great for the immune system)
- Anti-cancer
- Antispasmodic
- Expectorant
- Hypoalgesic (muscle pain)
- Blood thinner/increases circulation
- Osteoarthritis
- Lowers cholesterol
- Fever reducer, treats cold or flu
- Reduces nausea from motion sickness, pregnancy, etc
- Common cold symptoms including coughs
- Digestive problems
- Arthritis
- Migraines
- Hypertension

LAVENDAR

There have been multiple studies on the efficacy of lavender, and most have found it to be effective.

Older adults who drank lavender tea twice a day for two weeks in a small 2020 study experienced lower levels of anxiety and depression.

Other research indicates that several substances that help treat Alzheimer's - anticholinergic, neuroprotective, and antioxidant activities - are found in lavender.

Only the lavender buds are used for making tea. Add them to boiling water and brew for 10 minutes. Add a tablespoon of lavender buds for two cups of water - the longer you steep, the stronger the flavor. Once brewed, you can add honey or lemon flavor.

What it's good for:

- Antidepressant
- Antimicrobial
- Antioxidant
- Exhaustion
- Gentle sedative
- Hair Loss (alopecia aerata)
- Indigestion
- Imsomnia due to overactive mind
- Relaxation
- Relieves anxiety - nervousness and tension
- Relieves gas and bloating

MINT

While there isn't much scientific evidence for it working, many herbalists recommend peppermint oil for improving memory, and some studies have suggested it can help reduce asthma symptoms.

Peppermint has the most scientific evidence of being an effective cure for headaches. Two studies have found that peppermint oil can significantly reduce the severity of a tension headache within 15 minutes.

Peppermint essential oil has also been shown to reduce nausea - and can be particularly effective for seasickness, and there is evidence that Peppermint tea helps to treat constipation and a peppermint tea bag can be used to reduce the pain in your gums if you have a toothache.

For tea, add a cup of boiling water over dried mint and infuse for 10 minutes.

What it's good for:

- Anti-microbial (it was once added to milk to increase longevity)
- Anti-inflammatory
- Antioxidant - IBS and Constipation/intestinal spasms
- Calming
- Cramping
- Gas/bloating
- Menstral cramps
- Memory
- Nausea and vomiting
- Tension headaches
- Toothache (gums)

ROSEMARY

Rosemary is a great source of antioxidant phytonutrients. This includes flavonoids and carnosol, rosmanol, and rosmarinic acid (phenolic compounds). Rosmarinic acid has been shown to reduce inflammation and improve the action of liver enzymes responsible for metabolizing and detoxing our body.

Additionally, research has confirmed the historical claims of rosemary's memory stimulation abilities - breathing in rosemary's volatile oils helps enhance recall and increase alertness by stimulating the central nervous, respiratory, and motor systems.

Numerous studies also indicate that rosemary would prevent and limit some types of cancer progression.

Other validated medicinal uses of rosemary include antibacterial, anti-diabetic, anti-inflammatory, antinociceptive, antioxidant, antithrombotic, antiulcerogenic, antidiuretic, and hepatoprotective effects. And alcohol extract has shown an antidepressant effect.

As a tea, as well as having an anti-fungal effect, it can stimulate appetite and circulation, targeting blood supply to the abdominal organs, helping with the production of gastric and intestinal fluids, and improving skin circulation. It also has a strong antiseptic effect.

Here is a simple recipe for making rosemary tea:

Basic Rosemary Tea:

- Bring 1 cup of water to a boil.
- Remove from heat and add 1-2 sprigs of fresh rosemary.
- Cover and steep for 5-10 minutes.
- Remove the rosemary and sweeten with honey, if desired.

You can also add other herbs and spices to the tea, such as mint or ginger, to give it a different flavor.

What it's good for:

- Anti-bacterial
- Anti-fungal
- Antimicrobial

- Astringent
- Carminative (lessens intestinal gas)
- Cognition
- Anti-inflammatory
- Improve retention and recall facts
- Circulation
- Relieves aches and pains
- Improves eye health
- Regulates liver function
- Lower the risk of asthma

SAGE

Sage can lower cholesterol, rebuild vitality and strength weakened due to illness, and is a tonic for the liver.

Taking Sage by mouth has been shown to help improve memory and thinking skills, including memory loss and Alzheimer's disease. It does this by restoring the chemical balance in the brain. It is also used for reducing sweat, saliva, and depression.

It has been shown to improve the symptoms of menopause — particularly hot flushes, night sweats, and sleep problems.

It can also help reduce cholesterol and is often used to ease pain after surgery, for digestive problems (including loss of appetite and flatulence), stomach pain, diarrhea, bloating, and heartburn.

Although Sage is great for many illnesses, you need to be careful not to use it too high a dosage for a long time (using medicinal Sage for longer than two months). Some types of sage, including Common Sage, contain a chemical called Thujone, which can cause seizures, increase blood pressure, and may damage the liver and nervous system if consumed excessively. The amount of Thujone varies depending on the species of sage, when it was harvested, growing conditions, and other factors. Generally speaking, if you are using it in food, there are unlikely to be any side effects.

Sage tea is easy to make. Pour a cup of boiling water over a tablespoon of sage leaves, brew to the strength you like, then strain. You can add lemon, sugar, or honey to taste.

Add mint and cardamon pods to create a tea that eases nausea and stirs the appetite.

What it's good for:

- Anti-oxidant
- Anti-inflammatory
- Antiseptic
- Antimicrobial
- Improves memory and cognition
- Relieves mental lethargy and depression
- Cholesterol
- Symptoms of menopause
- Pain relief
- Stomach and digestion
- Sore throat (tea with honey and lemon)
- Fever
- Blood thinner
- Endocrine stabilizer/women's health
- Insomnia
- Excessive perspiration
- Libido stabilizer
- Treat older people with dryness of skin and hair

THYME

The most common variety of Thyme is Thymus vulgaris. It is well known as a medicinal plant, with flowers, leaves, and oils used to treat symptoms from diarrhea and stomach ache to arthritis.

Clinical studies have shown that thyme reduces coughing in people with bronchitis (it removes congestion) and can help with upper respiratory tract infections and common colds.

It can also increase the protective mucus layers in your stomach, which help protect the stomach lining from acid and is particularly good for liver function.

It has been found to protect against colon and breast cancer and help with fungal infections, including yeast infections.

People also use thyme to soothe coughing and manage hair loss (alopecia) and dementia.

It is considered safe when used in culinary amounts but check with a medical practitioner for medicinal uses, especially if you are taking other pharmaceutical drugs. Thyme may also slow blood clotting.

To make tea, just add a few sprigs to a cup of boiling water and let it brew for 5 to 20 minutes. You can add a twist of lemon for flavor.

<u>What it's good for:</u>

- Anti-oxidant
- Anti-bacterial
- Anti-inflammatory
- Anti-fungal
- Anti-infectious
- Anti-inflammatory

- Anti-microbial
- Anti-spasmodic
- Antiseptic (topical)
- Anti-viral
- Coughs - removes congestion (Fresh thyme is best)
- Food Preservative
- Improves immunity
- Enhances digestion

CHAPTER 7
Summary

I hope this short book is not only useful and practical so that you can get started right away, but I also hope that it has helped you understand which herbs to consider and why you should consider a particular herb in your tea.

Herbal tea really is simple to make and I have often been asked for various herbal tea suggestions for similar health problems - and it is the reason I decided to create this short book.

If you are not already using herbs, I hope that it has sparked your interest and that it might one day ignite a passion for these wonderful little green plants that we share our planet with.

This book was deliberately short and to the point because it really doesn't need to be long and involved and tea recipes don't need to be complicated.

Other than knowing which herbs to use, the biggest variation is steeping time (but this is also to taste). If you are using dried herbs then you will steep for a shorter time, while most fresh herbs take a bit longer. If I am using fresh herbs (like chamomile) I will often re-full the cup once or twice and leave the flower in the cup. If using the fresh leaves then you will tend to find that the small 'leaves' need strained. You can try the tea in a number of ways, so play with your timings and additions (honey, lemon, other herbs) to find the perfect tea for you.

You can also look into how the properties that these flavorings have can add even more to you tea. I tend to always use honey but love to use mint, cinnamon and lemon.

Thanks again for you interest and I hope you enjoy your herbal journey!

CHAPTER 8
Leave a review

Thank you for reading this book and I sincerely hope that you found it valuable. I would be eternally grateful if you would take just a few seconds to leave a review. You can leave a star rating or add some words.

So let me ask you this question. If it cost you nothing to share information with a struggling individual whom you don't personally know, would you do it? This person may have much in common with you, and this person, like most, judges a book by its reviews.

If you perceive this book as a valuable resource, would you take less than 60 seconds to leave an honest review? This act of kindness costs you nothing and could really help someone on their road to discovery. All with a review.

If you have enjoyed this book please follow the community page here https://www.facebook.com/GoldBerryHill

References

Understanding Herbal Remedies (Goldberry Hill)

Grow Your Own Medicinal Herbs (Goldberry Hill)

Discover the Power of Magic Tea (Goldberry Hill)

Friedrich, J., & logical, B. (2010. Green tea in dermatology. Journal of drugs in dermatology : JDD, 9(7), 753-759)

Thammaraks, K., & Asawanonda, P. (2012). Topical green tea extract for the treatment of acne vulgaris: a randomized, double-blind, controlled trial. International journal of dermatology, 51(12), 1480-1484)

Made in the USA
Las Vegas, NV
15 December 2023

82967972R00075